Practical Atlas of Transplant Pathology

W. Dean Wallace • Bita V. Naini

Editors

Practical Atlas of Transplant Pathology

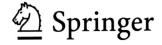
Springer

Editors
W. Dean Wallace
Department of Pathology and Laboratory
Medicine
David Geffen School of Medicine
at the University of California, Los Angeles
Los Angeles
CA
USA

Bita V. Naini
Department of Pathology and Laboratory
Medicine
David Geffen School of Medicine
at the University of California, Los Angeles
Los Angeles
CA
USA

ISBN 978-3-319-23053-5   ISBN 978-3-319-23054-2   (eBook)
DOI 10.1007/978-3-319-23054-2

Library of Congress Control Number: 2015954861

Springer Cham Heidelberg New York Dordrecht London

Springer International Publishing AG Switzerland is part of Springer Science+Business Media (www.springer.com)

It is with great appreciation and affection that we acknowledge our teachers in transplant pathology: Galen Cortina, Michael Fishbein, and Charlie Lassman.

Preface

It has been said, "The most important tool for the pathologist is the telephone, not the microscope." This might be a little tongue in cheek, but it does point to a fundamental truth about the practice of pathology; our ability to communicate effectively with our clinical colleagues does not just inform our diagnostic interpretations and enable us to deliver more accurate diagnoses, but is absolutely necessary to be able to practice at the standard of care our patients deserve. No area of pathology is more reliant on close interactions between clinicians and pathologist than transplant pathology to make the correct diagnosis; in few other areas are the results as critical and time-sensitive as in the transplant setting. While morphologic assessment remains the primary function of anatomic pathology, it cannot be overemphasized that recognition of the morphologic pattern of injury is often only one important step in solving the puzzle of allograft dysfunction. The assimilation of biopsy findings with clinical, laboratory, and imaging findings may ultimately be needed to establish the underlying etiology of the allograft dysfunction.

This book is partly based on the experience and practice of the pathologists at UCLA, one of the world's busiest and most comprehensive transplant centers. While our group's collective experience is vast, we are, of course, massively indebted to our colleagues at transplant centers around the world for their contributions to the literature and understanding of transplant pathology. No man, or transplant center, is an island.

This book is divided into different chapters based on transplanted organ as well as two additional chapters devoted to the review of transplant immunogenetics (Chap. 1) and post-transplant lymphoproliferative disorders (Chap. 9). These chapters are intended to provide additional information that may aid the practicing pathologist to understand the pathophysiology of transplant rejection and assist in the evaluation of lymphomatous transformation in the transplant setting. The organ-specific chapters discuss the diagnostic criteria for rejection as well as outlining the most common causes of allograft dysfunction for each organ. However, the emphasis is meant to be on the many images provided that depict the most common morphologic findings seen in each organ in the transplant setting. An appendix is also provided which includes information such as the UCLA protocols used in processing biopsies as well as sample templates for reporting allograft biopsy interpretations.

We hope this atlas will serve as a practical tool not just for transplant pathologists but also general pathologists who are increasingly confronted with allograft-related problems which may occur when transplant-recipient patients show up at their institutions, seemingly out of the blue. If you find yourself struggling over a difficult biopsy, as we all do from time to time, you may find your telephone to be just as helpful as your microscope.

Los Angeles, CA, USA

W. Dean Wallace
Bita V. Naini

Acknowledgments

We would like to sincerely thank the contributing authors for sharing their expertise and adding greatly to the quality of this book and Leslie Chew for assistance with preparation of the manuscript. We also gratefully acknowledge the assistance of Lee Klein and Joanna Bolesworth from Springer for their support throughout this project and for making this book possible.

Contents

Contributors

Kourosh Beroukhim, BS David Geffen School of Medicine at the University of California, Los Angeles, Los Angeles, CA, USA

J. Michael Cecka, PhD Department of Pathology and Laboratory Medicine, David Geffen School of Medicine at the University of California, Los Angeles, Los Angeles, CA, USA

M. Fernando Palma Diaz, MD Department of Pathology and Laboratory Medicine, David Geffen School of Medicine at the University of California, Los Angeles, Los Angeles, CA, USA

Carol Farver, MD Pathology and Laboratory Medicine Institute, Cleveland Clinic, Cleveland, OH, USA

Michael C. Fishbein, MD Department of Pathology and Laboratory Medicine, David Geffen School of Medicine at the University of California, Los Angeles, Los Angeles, CA, USA

Samuel W. French, MD, PhD Department of Pathology and Laboratory Medicine, David Geffen School of Medicine at the University of California, Los Angeles, Los Angeles, CA, USA

Michelle J. Hickey, PhD Department of Pathology and Laboratory Medicine, David Geffen School of Medicine at the University of California, Los Angeles, Los Angeles, CA, USA

Jamie Koo, MD Department of Pathology and Laboratory Medicine, David Geffen School of Medicine at the University of California, Los Angeles, Los Angeles, CA, USA

James H. Lan, PhD Department of Pathology and Laboratory Medicine, David Geffen School of Medicine at the University of California, Los Angeles, Los Angeles, CA, USA

Charles R. Lassman, MD, PhD Department of Pathology and Laboratory Medicine, David Geffen School of Medicine at the University of California, Los Angeles, Los Angeles, CA, USA

Bita V. Naini, MD Department of Pathology and Laboratory Medicine, David Geffen School of Medicine at the University of California, Los Angeles, Los Angeles, CA, USA

Elaine F. Reed, MD Department of Pathology and Laboratory Medicine, David Geffen School of Medicine at the University of California, Los Angeles, Los Angeles, CA, USA

Jonathan Said, MD Department of Pathology and Laboratory Medicine, David Geffen School of Medicine at the University of California, Los Angeles, Los Angeles, CA, USA

Chandra Smart, MD Department of Pathology and Laboratory Medicine, David Geffen School of Medicine at the University of California, Los Angeles, Los Angeles, CA, USA

Eric A. Swanson, MD Department of Pathology and Laboratory Medicine, David Geffen School of Medicine at the University of California, Los Angeles, Los Angeles, CA, USA

Nicole M. Valenzuela, PhD Department of Pathology and Laboratory Medicine, David Geffen School of Medicine at the University of California, Los Angeles, Los Angeles, CA, USA

W. Dean Wallace, MD Department of Pathology and Laboratory Medicine, David Geffen School of Medicine at the University of California, Los Angeles, Los Angeles, CA, USA

Hanlin L. Wang, MD, PhD Department of Pathology and Laboratory Medicine, David Geffen School of Medicine at the University of California, Los Angeles, Los Angeles, CA, USA

Qiuheng Zhang, PhD Department of Pathology and Laboratory Medicine, David Geffen School of Medicine at the University of California, Los Angeles, Los Angeles, CA, USA

Xiaohai Zhang, PhD Department of Pathology and Laboratory Medicine, David Geffen School of Medicine at the University of California, Los Angeles, Los Angeles, CA, USA

Jonathan E. Zuckerman, MD, PhD Department of Pathology and Laboratory Medicine, David Geffen School of Medicine at the University of California, Los Angeles, CA, USA

Histocompatibility and Immunogenetics for Solid Organ Transplantation

Qiuheng Zhang, Michelle J. Hickey, Nicole M. Valenzuela, Xiaohai Zhang, James H. Lan, J. Michael Cecka, and Elaine F. Reed

Disparity of human leukocyte antigen (HLA) molecules between a transplant recipient and a donor elicits the generation of alloreactive T and B cells that mediate graft rejection. Matching HLA of the donor and recipient reduces alloreactivity and prolongs graft survival in organ transplants. However, only few transplants are actually performed between HLA-identical individuals, and life-long immunosuppression is needed to prevent graft rejection. Accurate assessment of immunological risk factors coupled with precise tools for diagnosis and classification of rejection is critical for successful treatment and prevention of rejection. HLA testing has evolved substantially over the last 50 years with the advent of comprehensive molecular HLA typing and sensitive solid-phase HLA antibody identification assays that enable new strategies for donor-recipient risk assessment. This chapter provides an overview of the HLA system and mechanisms underlying allograft rejection. We also discuss the diagnostic tests performed by the Immunogenetics Laboratory to assess risk, diagnose transplant rejection, and guide immunosuppressive therapy.

Q. Zhang, PhD • M.J. Hickey, PhD • N.M. Valenzuela, PhD
X. Zhang, PhD • J.H. Lan, PhD • J.M. Cecka, PhD
E.F. Reed, MD (✉)
Department of Pathology and Laboratory Medicine,
David Geffen School of Medicine at the University of California,
Los Angeles, Los Angeles, CA, USA
e-mail: ereed@mednet.ucla.edu

1.1 Structure and Function of HLA

1.1.1 Genomic Organization, Structure, and Function of HLA

The human major histocompatibility complex (MHC) region on chromosome 6 is composed of highly polymorphic HLA class I genes (HLA-A, -B, -C), HLA class II genes (HLA-DR, -DQ, -DP), nonclassical class I genes (HLA-E, -F, -G), and class I–like genes (MICA, MICB) (Fig. 1.1a) [1, 2]. The key functions of HLA class I molecules are presentation of intracellular peptide antigens to CD8+ T lymphocytes and serving as ligands of receptors on natural killer (NK) cells. The nonclassical HLA-E and HLA-G proteins also serve as ligands for NK cell receptors to generate inhibitory signals that prevent NK cells from eliciting cell killing. Conversely, the stress-induced MICA and MICB antigens expressed by activated T cells, endothelial cells, gut, and transformed cells bind NKG2D receptors and activate NK cell immune responses and cell killing. The HLA class II antigens play an important role in antigen presentation to CD4+ T cells.

The HLA-DR genomic region contains one functional gene for the α-chain (DRA), which pairs with one or two functional genes for the β-chain (DRB1, DRB3, DRB4, DRB5) resulting in expression of the DR51, DR52, or DR53 antigens depending on the HLA-DRB1 allele type (Fig. 1.1b) [1, 2]. The HLA class III region, between the genes for class I and class II on chromosome 6, contains many immune genes involved in immune function including complement and cytokine genes (Fig. 1.1a).

Structurally, the HLA class I molecule is a heterodimer consisting of a heavy α chain that is bound noncovalently to β_2-microglobulin (β_2m) light chain, a non-MHC gene (located in chromosome 15) (Fig. 1.2). The HLA class II molecule is composed of two transmembrane glycoprotein chains, α (encoded by DRA, DQA1, or DPA1) and β (encoded by DRB, DQB1, or DPB1). Each chain has two domains, and the α_1 and β_1 domains of class II molecules form the peptide-binding cleft. The pockets located in the groove accommodate distinct peptides with specific characteristics (Fig. 1.2). Therefore, each HLA binds different peptides.

The T-cell receptor recognizes self-HLA molecules containing a peptide fragment to elicit an immune response.

In the setting of allotransplantation, the patient's T-cell receptors can recognize intact donor HLA molecules through a pathway called "direct" allorecognition as described later.

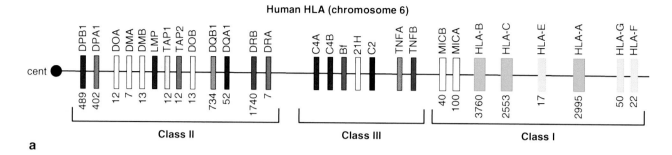

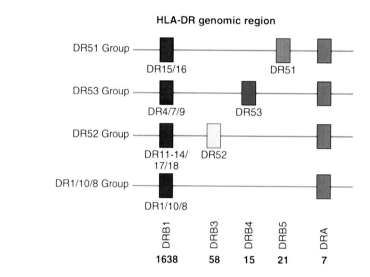

Fig. 1.1 Genetic map of the human and mouse MHCs. (**a**) Schematic map of human MHC on chromosome 6. Illustrations are not drawn to scale. The centromere (*circle*) and major HLA are indicated in order. The number of distinct proteins (alleles) encoded by each human MHC gene is indicated under each locus. (**b**) Based on the DRB1 allele type, human MHC haplotypes fall into four groups—DR51, DR52, DR53, and DR1/10/8—that vary in *DRB* gene number. The serological specificities encoded by each *DRB* gene are provided underneath each locus (loci are indicated by *boxes*). The number of alleles encoded by each *DRB* gene is indicated. (**a**, *Data* from IMGT/HLA database, release 3.19; http://www.ebi.ac.uk/imgt/hla/stats.html [1, 2]; **b**, Data from IMGT/HLA database, January 2015; http://www.ebi.ac.uk/imgt/hla/stats.html [1, 2])

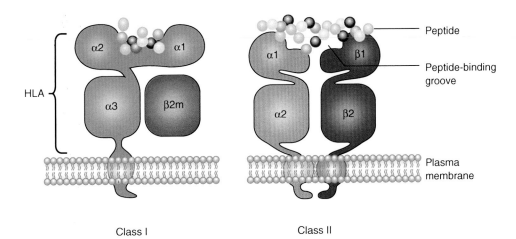

Class I   Class II

Fig. 1.2 Structure of HLA molecules. HLA class I and class II molecules present peptide antigens to CD8+ and CD4+ T cells, respectively. The HLA class I molecule is a heterodimer of a membrane-spanning heavy α chain (encoded by HLA-A, -B, or –C gene) bound noncovalently to a non-MHC gene (located in chromosome 15)–encoded light β2-microglobulin (β2m) chain, which does not span the membrane. The α chain folds into three domains: α1, α2, and α3. The α1 and α2 domains form the antigen-binding groove. The HLA class II molecule is composed of two transmembrane glycoprotein chains, α (encoded by DRA, DQA1 or DPA1) and β (encoded by DRB1, DQB1 or DPB1). Each chain has two domains, and the two chains together form a compact four-domain structure similar to that of a HLA class I molecule. The α2 and β2 domains, like the α3- and β2-microglobulin domains of the HLA class I molecule, have amino acid sequence and structural similarities to IgC domains. The α1 and β1 domains of class II molecules form the peptide-binding cleft. The major difference between class I and class II is that the ends of the peptide-binding groove are more open in HLA class II molecules than in HLA class I molecules. As a result, the HLA class I can accommodate only short peptides (~9 amino acids long) and the ends of the peptide are substantially buried within the class I molecule. In contrast, the class II groove has open ends and can accommodate longer peptides (12–20 amino acids long)

1.1.2 HLA Gene Polymorphism, Haplotypes, and Inheritance

The most notable feature of the human MHC is the remarkable degree of polymorphism. To date, over 9400 distinct HLA class I alleles and 3000 class II alleles have been recognized [1]. The polymorphic regions are principally localized to the amino terminal region of these molecules, which bind peptides and interact with T-cell receptors. Although the high degree of HLA polymorphism is necessary for enhancing the diversity in the repertoire of HLA-bound peptides to combat pathogens, it creates a significant barrier for transplantation of histoincompatible tissues and organs between individuals.

The collection of MHC alleles present on each parental chromosome is called an HLA haplotype. HLAs are inherited in Mendelian fashion, which means that each parental chromosome 6 provides a haplotype or linked set of MHC genes to the offspring. A child is a one-haplotype match to each parent unless recombination, or a "crossover," between genes of the parental haplotype occurs. Statistically, there is a 25 % chance that siblings will share the same parental haplotypes (HLA-identical), a 50 % chance they will share one haplotype (one-haplotype match), and a 25 % chance that neither haplotype will be the same (zero-haplotype match) (Fig. 1.3).

Box 1.1

The HLA region demonstrates strong linkage disequilibrium across HLA-A, -B, -C, -DR, -DQ, and -DP alleles. Linkage disequilibrium is a phenomenon in which alleles at adjacent HLA loci are inherited together more often than would be expected by chance. Existing data suggest that positive selection is operating on the haplotype and that the linked loci confer a particular selective advantage for the host.

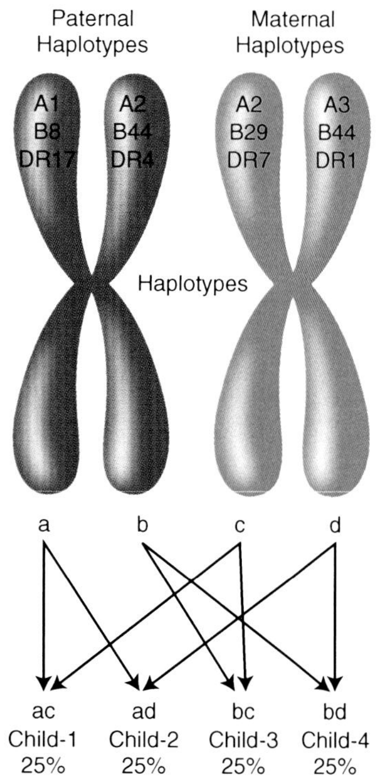

Fig. 1.3 HLA haplotype segregation in a family. Each child inherits one HLA haplotype from each parent. Because each parent has two different haplotypes (paternal = ab and maternal = cd), four different haplotypic combinations are possible in the offspring (ac, ad, bc, bd). Therefore, a child has a 25 % chance of having an HLA-identical– or zero-haplotype–matched sibling donor, and a 50 % chance of having a one-haplotype–matched sibling donor. All children have one-haplotype matched to each parent unless recombination has occurred

1.1.3 HLA Matching for Solid Organ Transplantation

Prior to transplant, recipients and donors are HLA-typed and mismatched antigens are identified. It is well established that renal transplants from HLA-identical sibling donors survive 50 % longer on average than transplants from HLA-mismatched living donors [3]. Similarly, kidney grafts from deceased donors that have no HLA-A, -B, or -DR locus antigen mismatches survive longer than grafts from donors carrying HLA mismatches. In order to increase the number of HLA-matched transplants, the degree of HLA compatibility has been incorporated into deceased donor kidney allocation systems in many countries. However, given the extensive polymorphism of the HLA system, grafts carrying similar HLA genotypes from unrelated donors are uncommon. HLA matching is, therefore, not considered in the allocation of most solid organ transplants except for national sharing of HLA-matched renal allografts for highly sensitized recipients and HLA-DR matching allocation of locally procured kidneys.

1.1.4 Cellular Responses to HLA Alloantigens

Allorecognition is the activation of the transplant recipient's adaptive immune response to mismatched donor histocompatibility antigens following transplant [4, 5]. Activation of the recipient's CD4+ T lymphocytes is a pivotal step in the initiation of the immune response to alloantigens following transplantation leading to downstream activation of cytotoxic CD8+ T lymphocytes and antibody-producing B cells. Evidence supports three mechanisms of allorecognition: the direct, indirect, and semidirect pathways (Fig. 1.4). These pathways of allorecognition can occur independently or simultaneously and are associated with graft pathology and transplant outcome.

The direct pathway is the activation of the transplant recipient's CD4+ and CD8+ T cells by HLA:peptide complexes on the surface of donor cells that are transplanted as passengers with the organ. The donor's antigen presenting cells (APCs), expressing foreign HLA, migrate to the secondary lymph nodes of the recipient and present donor antigens to the recipient's CD4+ T cells. The strength of the immune response elicited by the direct allorecognition pathway correlates to the high frequency of recipient allogeneic T cells that become activated during the first few weeks following transplant, mediating acute rejection. CD4+ T cells activated through the direct pathway are capable of providing help to effector CD8+ T cells, therefore promoting cell-mediated rejection of the transplanted organ (Fig. 1.4).

In contrast to the direct allorecognition pathway, indirect allorecognition is the activation of the transplant recipient's CD4+ T cells by alloantigen that is processed and presented in the context of the recipient's HLA. Donor antigens, shed by the grafted organ, are processed and presented in the context of self-restricted HLA class II by the recipient's B cells. The recipient's follicular helper CD4+ T cells are then activated to provide help, leading to the generation of alloreactive CD8+ effector T cells and antibody-producing B cells (Fig. 1.4). The immune response engendered by this pathway can incite cell-mediated or antibody-mediated rejection and is credited with driving chronic rejection. Also, owing to the lower frequency of T cells with indirect allospecificity, and requirements for antigen processing, the indirect pathway is physiodynamically slower than the response to presentation through the direct pathway. It usually takes 14 days for de novo donor-specific antibodies (DSAs) to develop after transplantation.

The semidirect pathway of allorecognition is presented as a hypothesis to describe events of apparent overlap between the direct and the indirect pathways from animal models of transplant rejection indicating that indirectly activated allospecific CD4+ T cells can provide help to directly activated allospecific CD8+ T cells [6]. The mechanism underling the phenomenon of semidirect allorecognition likely lies in the exchange of membrane proteins between immune cells. After transplantation, the recipient's dendritic cells (DCs) acquire intact donor HLA class I:peptide complexes from donor passenger DC or endothelial cells either through membrane exchange or by uptake of exosomes, or vesicles, containing the antigen that are shed from donor tissue. The recipient's DC then bears intact donor HLA class I molecules as well as recipient HLA class II molecules, and is capable of stimulating the recipient's CD4+ and CD8+ T cells via the indirect and direct pathways (Fig. 1.4).

Box 1.2

Common in vitro assays used to measure direct and indirect alloreactivity include the mixed lymphocyte culture (MLR), cytotoxic precursor T-cell assay, cytokine ELISPOT, or flow cytometry. To measure alloactivation via the direct allorecognition pathway, recipient T cells are cocultured with irradiated/inactivated donor APCs. For the indirect allorecognition pathway, recipient T cells are cocultured with autologous APCs pulsed with donor cellular protein fragments, or synthetic peptides.

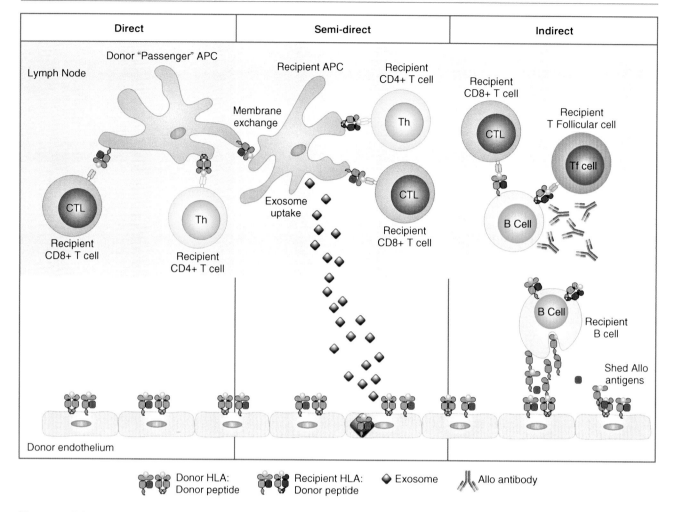

Fig. 1.4 Alloimmune responses occur through direct, indirect, and semidirect recognition. The direct pathway involves presentation of allogeneic MHC class I and II antigens on donor APCs to recipient CD4+ and cytotoxic CD8+ T cells (*CTL*) and is believed to be the primary mechanism of acute rejection. The indirect pathway involves processing the donor alloantigens by recipient B cells and presentation to recipient T-follicular cells and CTL. Alloantibodies are generated by interaction of alloreactive B cells with CD4+ T cells, and can lead to AMR. The indirect recognition pathway is considered a major pathway mediating chronic rejection. In the semidirect pathway, intact donor HLA class I:peptide complexes are presented on the DC of the recipient (through either membrane exchange or exosome uptake) to recipient CD8+ T cells. Simultaneously, processed donor peptide is presented in the context of the recipient's HLA class II to the recipient's CD4+ T cells. The recipient's T-helper cells, activated by the indirect pathway, can then provide "help" to the recipient's CTL, activated by the direct pathway. *Blue* indicates donor HLA class I and II. *Purple* indicates recipient HLA class I and II

1.1.5 HLA Typing

HLA antigens were initially defined using serological microlymphocytotoxicity techniques that used a battery of carefully selected antisera to recognize distinct HLAs on the surface of lymphocytes. During the past 20 years, more precise DNA-based typing techniques have replaced serological methods in clinical applications. The three basic DNA-based HLA typing techniques used in conjunction with polymerase chain reaction (PCR) are the reverse sequence-specific oligonucleotide (rSSO) probe hybridization method, sequence-specific primer (SSP) directed amplification method, and sequencing-based typing (SBT) method. The basic premise for these assays is that the HLA genes are selectively amplified by the PCR followed by detection of the specific polymorphisms by gel electrophoretic mobility (SSP) (Fig. 1.5a), direct DNA sequencing (SBT), or hybridization with sequence-specific oligonucleotide probes (rSSO) (Fig. 1.5b).

Development of rapid, high-throughput sequencing and PCR assays for HLA typing have allowed for a more accurate definition of recipient and donor HLA genotypes. High-resolution HLA typing, which is achieved by SBT, allows for differentiation of unique epitopes to which a recipient may make specific antibodies. One major limitation of SBT is that it often results in ambiguous typing due to the sharing of nucleotide sequences across the specific exons interrogated and additional testing is required to report the allele-level typing results. Implementation of next-generation sequencing (NGS) technologies should eliminate the problem of HLA genotyping ambiguities. The NGS technology enables parallel sequencing of billions of PCR-amplified DNA fragments. Many groups have developed long-range PCR strategies to amplify the full length of the HLA genes, followed by fragmentation of the amplified DNA, and sequencing by NGS. Coupling the NGS strategy with sophisticated software algorithms to perform the assembly of the sequenced fragments provides in-phase, full-length allele-level typing.

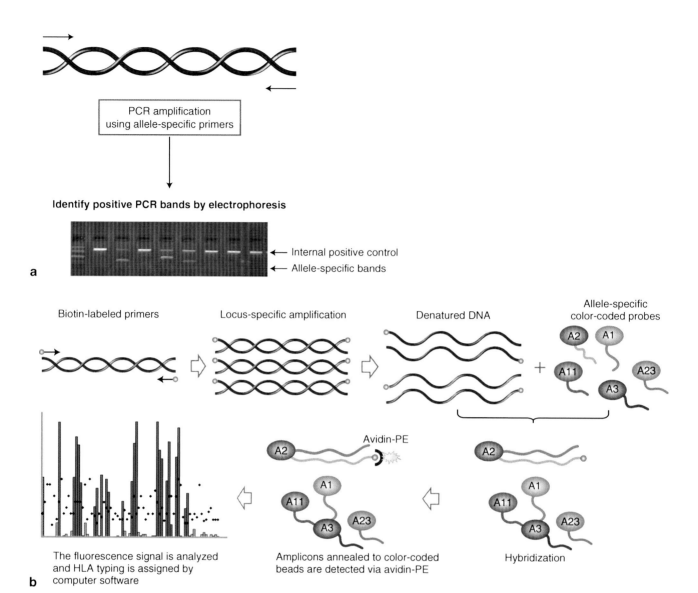

Fig. 1.5 Molecular HLA typing. (**a**) HLA typing by SSP. Each PCR well contains a unique set of primers that are designed to have perfect matches with a single allele or group of alleles and produce a product with a particular known size. A picture of an agarose gel electrophoresis shows the pattern of allele-/group-specific PCR products corresponding to amplification of HLA class I or class II genes. Under strictly controlled PCR conditions, perfectly matched primer pairs result in the amplification of target sequences and an identifiable band on an agarose gel (i.e., a positive reaction) whereas mismatched primer pairs do not amplify (i.e., a negative reaction). Each PCR reaction also includes a positive internal control primer pair that amplifies a conserved gene segment (i.e., human β-globulin gene), which is present in all human DNA samples and is used to verify the integrity of the PCR reaction. (**b**) The reverse single-nucleotide probe hybridization (SSOP) method using Luminex bead arrays. DNA samples are PCR-amplified using biotin-conjugated locus-specific primers. The PCR products are denatured and hybridized with probe arrays of Luminex color-coded polystyrene beads. Amplicons annealed to the polystyrene beads are detected via streptavidin phycoerythrin (*PE*) chemistry. Fluorescence signals of both PE and color-coded beads are detected by using the Luminex 100 flow-based instrument. The combined data are analyzed and HLA typing is assigned by a software program

1.2 Role of HLA Antibodies in Transplantation

Sensitization to non-self HLA through pregnancies, prior transplantation, and/or blood transfusions increases the risk of allograft rejection and limits the patient's access to organ transplantation. The Organ Procurement Transplant Network data indicate as many as 30 % of patients waiting for transplantation are presensitized to HLA antigens. Circulating DSAs in a transplant candidate may damage the graft to varying degrees depending on the DSA titer, specificity, and level of HLAs expression on the graft. High-titered pre-transplant DSA directed against HLA class I antigens can cause catastrophic hyperacute rejection and immediate graft loss, whereas high-titer class II DSAs mediate graft rejection 2–4 days after transplant, upon re-expression of HLA class II antigens on the endothelium of the allograft. In contrast, pre-transplant DSAs of low titer are often associated with development of acute antibody-mediated rejection (AMR) during the first 3 months after transplantation. If left untreated, patients with AMR are at risk of graft loss and/or markedly shortened overall graft survival time. Patients producing de novo anti-HLA antibodies against their donor following transplantation are also at increased risk of graft failure unless their response can be controlled or abrogated. The effect of post-transplant DSAs on different transplanted organs may differ in acute severity, in the specific pathological lesions, and ultimately, the degree of damage they cause to the organ, but evidence is rapidly accruing that shows these antibodies can damage any transplanted organ including kidney, heart, lung, intestine, and liver. Standard treatment for AMR consists of repeated plasmapheresis, immunoadsorption, intravenous immune globulin (IVIG), splenectomy, and eculizumab. Various combinations of these therapeutic modalities have been successfully used to treat AMR and improve outcomes in some patients; however, in many cases, interventions for AMRs are not always effective.

1.2.1 Antibody Biology

Human immunoglobulins are divided into 5 isotypes (IgM, IgD, IgG, IgE, and IgA). IgG and IgA are further subdivided into several subclasses each (IgG1, IgG2, IgG3, and IgG4; and IgA1 and IgA2). Antibody isotype and subclass are important determinants of both affinity for antigen and capacity to trigger immune effector functions. Antibody structure, complement-fixing capacity, and affinity for Fc receptors (FcγRs) is illustrated in Fig. 1.6. IgG is the predominant isotype in circulation, and although antibodies to HLA may be IgM, IgA, or IgG, clinical studies to date have concluded that IgG to donor HLA is most clinically relevant, although recent evidence points to a pathogenic effect of persistent IgM.

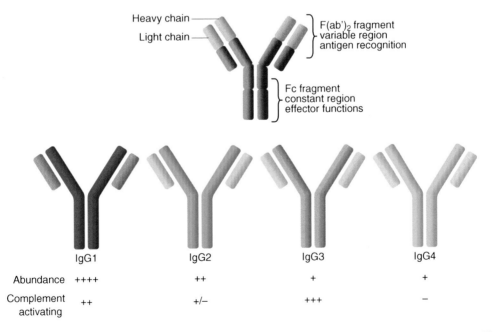

Fig. 1.6 Antibody structure and biology. Human immunoglobulin is composed of a light chain and a heavy chain, each of which contains a constant region and a variable region. The variable regions of the light and heavy chains combine to form the three-dimensional antigen-binding region. The constant region of the heavy chain forms the Fc fragment, which interacts with immune effector systems, including complement and innate immune cell Fc receptors. The predominant isotype in circulation is IgG, which consists of four subclasses—IgG1, IgG2, IgG3, and IgG4—numbered in order of their relative abundance in circulation. Each subclass has different constant regions and, therefore, a different capacity to elicit Fc-mediated functions, including activating of complement

1.2.2 Antibody Effector Functions

Recognition of antigen by the F(ab')₂ fragment elicits cross-linking of the target HLA and triggers activation of intracellular signaling cascades, described later (see Sect. 1.2.8). In addition, antibodies carry out their canonical effector functions through the Fc fragment, which bridges innate effector systems with adaptive immunity. Antibodies can activate the classical complement cascade to trigger production of soluble and cell-bound inflammatory mediators and can interact with receptors on myeloid and innate lymphoid cells to mediate cellular functions [7]. Both of these functions are reflected in the diagnostic criteria of AMR in kidney and heart allografts, manifesting as C4d deposition in the microvasculature and intravascular macrophage (CD68) or neutrophil infiltration in the allograft. In the following section, we briefly review the biology of the complement system and discuss the implications and limitations to the current use of markers of these processes in the pathological diagnosis of AMR.

1.2.3 Complement

With the recognition that antibodies to donor HLA can cause rejection in renal allografts came the need for accurate pathological markers of AMR. Detection of classical complement activation in renal allografts in regraft patients. In recipients with circulating antibodies and intense C3d and C4d deposition in peritubular capillaries was first reported in the early 1990s. The current diagnostic criteria for AMR in cardiac, renal, and pancreas allografts include immunohistochemical staining for C4d, as a pathological marker of activation of the complement cascade in the microvasculature. Although microvascular C4d alone is not a specific indicator of AMR, in conjunction with other pathological evidence of antibody-mediated injury, it has important utility in kidney, heart, and pancreas allografts. However, in other solid organs, including lung, liver, and small bowel, the clinical utility of C4d is unclear and currently no consensus criteria for the pathologic diagnosis of AMR exist. In order to understand why C4d is pathologically significant, why it may not always specifically indicate rejection, and why it may have variable utility among organs, it is necessary to briefly review the complement cascade.

1.2.3.1 What Is C4d?

Complement is an ancient system of innate immunity composed of circulating plasma proteins. Complement becomes activated at sites of inflammation to tag pathogens or dysfunctional host cells for destruction by facilitating opsonization, promoting recruitment of immune effector cells, and causing direct lysis of gram-negative bacteria, fungi, enveloped viruses, and antibody-coated host cells. Inactive under quiescent conditions, complement proteins include zymogens, which are activated upon cleavage and, through a series of catalytic events, generate inflammatory split products [8].

Complement activation proceeds stepwise from recognition of target surfaces, which triggers activation of catalytic complement proteins that successively cleave their targets (Fig. 1.7). The peptide products of cleavage form active convertases that cleave other complement proteins or inflammatory mediators called anaphylatoxins and opsonins. Terminal complement activation may cause lysis of the target cell, a phenomenon called complement-dependent cytotoxicity (CDC). However, host cells express a variety of cell surface complement regulatory receptors, and several complement inhibitory proteins are also present in the circulation. At each step, these soluble and membrane-bound host regulatory proteins degrade active complement components to restrict the magnitude, location, and duration of complement-mediated damage. For complement activation, particularly lysis, to occur at the surface of the host cell, it must exceed the threshold set by negative regulation by endogenous complement inhibitors. CDC resulting in cell death is, therefore, thought to be an exceptional event observed under conditions of extreme complement activation, such as during hyperacute rejection.

Three pathways of complement are defined by the distinct mechanisms of initiation, although ultimately these pathways converge on the same downstream actors. The alternative complement pathway is activated directly at the cell surface of pathogens by deposition of spontaneously generated C3b and advances to terminal complement activation owing to the lack of inhibitory molecules on microbial surfaces. The lectin pathway also targets pathogens through specific recognition of microbial carbohydrate. Lastly, the classical pathway is activated by antibody bound to the surface of target cells, linking complement to adaptive immunity. Here, antibody is recognized by complement C1 complex that binds to the Fc region of certain isotypes and subclasses of immunoglobulin. It is this pathway that is thought to lie at the heart of HLA antibody–mediated allograft injury and rejection.

The classical complement pathway is initiated by IgM or certain subclasses of IgG binding to antigens on target cells, which are recognized by the C1q subunit of the C1 complex. The globular heads of C1q bridge the proximal Fc tails of antigen-complexed antibody. The capacity of an antibody to bind to C1q and elicit complement activation is dependent upon several independent factors, including antibody subclass, affinity, titer, and glycosylation. Binding of C1q to HLA antibodies can be detected in vitro using C1qScreen assay (Fig. 1.7). DSAs that bind C1q in this assay are predicted to activate the complement cascade (e.g., distinguishing the effective complement activator IgG3 from the relatively inactive IgG4). To date, the reports of the prognostic value of this assay have been somewhat variable, and more work is needed to elucidate its utility in predicting outcome.

> **Box 1.3**
> Complement C1 complex binding to antibody through C1q induces a conformation change in the catalytic subunit C1r. C1r then cleaves C1s to activate its serine protease function. Activated C1s is capable of cleaving C4 into C4a and C4b, the latter of which covalently attaches to the target surface near C1. Whereas C4a remains soluble and acts as an anaphylatoxin, C4b can either complex with a split product of C2 (C2a) generated by C1s to form an active convertase or be disabled by complement regulatory proteins. Uncleaved C4b in complex with C2a forms the C3 convertase, which cleaves C3 into soluble inflammatory C3a, and the immobilized opsonin C3b, which joins with C4bC2a to form the C5 convertase. Catalysis of C5 by this complex causes terminal complement activation, generating the potent anaphylatoxin C5a and the peptide C5b. C5b initiates formation of the MAC by recruiting C6, C7, C8, and C9. The MAC forms a pore that penetrates the target cell membrane and, at high concentrations, may cause lysis, a final outcome that is measured in the complement-dependent cytotoxicity crossmatch (CDC-XM) assay.

C1q:antibody binding triggers a complex cascade of cleavage events, producing soluble inflammatory mediators such as C3a and C5a, and cell surface–associated products including the membrane attack complex (MAC). The MAC forms a pore that penetrates the target cell membrane and may cause lysis. The potential for HLA antibodies to damage prospective donor cells through MAC formation is measured in the clinical test called complement-dependent cytotoxicity crossmatch (CDC-XM), discussed in more detail later (see Sect. 1.2.4). Notably, C5 cleavage is inhibited by the drug eculizumab, preventing production of C5a and formation of MAC.

Several complement split products remain covalently linked to the target cell membrane and can be detected immunohistologically. C4d is thus far the most useful of these for the diagnosis of AMR. It is generated from degradation of C4b by negative regulators (C4b-binding protein, complement receptor 1 [CR1], membrane cofactor protein [MCP, CD46], or Factor I), which release a C4c peptide and reveal the small C4d split product. C4d remains covalently linked to the cell membrane and has a longer half-life than C4b because of this turnover mechanism. Its immunohistological detection in the microvasculature indicates early activation of the complement cascade, specifically marking cleavage of C4. C3b is similarly regulated by inhibitory proteins, and its degradation is marked at the cell surface by C3d. In vitro assays measuring C3d generation by HLA antibodies in vitro may have added utility compared with C1qScreen, because C3d is much further downstream than C1q and this assay is functionally dependent upon physiological activation of complement (Fig. 1.7).

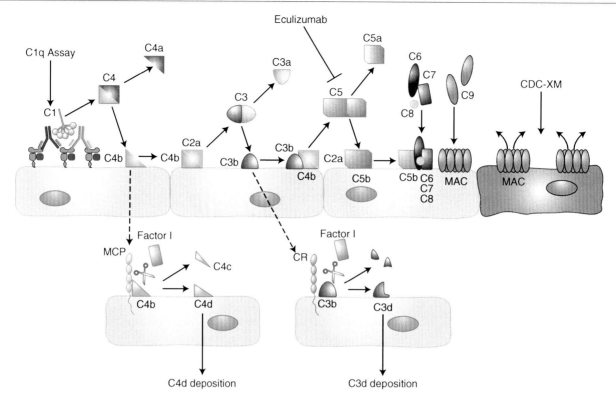

Fig. 1.7 The classical complement cascade. Antibody binding to antigen, in this case, to HLA class I on donor endothelial cells, in close proximity permits binding of the C1 complex and initiation of the classical complement cascade. The C1q assay measures the binding of HLA antibodies to C1q (a component of the C1 complex) on single-antigen beads. The C1 complex cleaves C4 to generate C4b. Catalytic products such as C4b can go on to form convertases and soluble mediators that perpetuate and amplify the complement cascade (*solid arrows*) or can be targeted by endogenous inhibitors to inactivate them (*dashed arrows*). For example, C4b either combines with C2a to form a catalytically active complex to cleave C3 or is degraded by complement regulatory proteins and inhibitors such as MCP and Factor I (*dashed line*), to

generate C4d. C4d remains covalently linked to the cell membrane and is a marker of early complement activation. Cleavage of C3 generates the inflammatory product C3a and the cell surface–bound C3b. Like C4b, C3b can either be degraded by inhibitory proteins (complement receptors 1–3 and Factor I) to yield C3d or form a catalytic complex, with the C4b/C2a complex, that acts on C5. When C5 is cleaved, soluble C5a, a potent anaphylatoxin, and C5b are generated. Eculizumab is an anti-C5 antibody that binds to C5 with very high affinity and prevents its cleavage. C5b recruits several other complement proteins to the cell surface and ultimately promotes the formation of the MAC. MAC forms pores in the cell membrane and, at high levels, can cause lysis of the cell. This outcome is measured in the CDC-XM assay (Fig. 1.8)

1.2.3.2 Why Might C4d Not Be Specific?

It is important to note that C4d is relatively far upstream in the classical complement cascade. Therefore, detection of C4d does not guarantee downstream terminal complement activation that leads to anaphylatoxin production or cell lysis (MAC). Indeed many regulatory checkpoints downstream of C4 prevent this in most cases, and endothelial cells are quite resistant to complement-dependent lysis in vitro. Interestingly, in C4d-positive cardiac biopsies, concurrent expression of the complement inhibitors decay accelerating factor (DAF), CD55, and CD59 on endothelium were increased in patients without allograft dysfunction but absent in those with impairment [9, 10]. These and other results suggest that, despite evidence of C4d deposition and early complement activation, endogenous complement inhibitory proteins may protect the allograft from damage during AMR. It has been suggested that immunohistological detection of C3d, which is counterintuitively downstream of C4d (Fig. 1.7), might be a superior indicator of more advanced complement activation [10].

In addition, clinically relevant HLA antibodies are of the IgG isotype. Blood group disparities are recognized by natural IgM, a potent activator of the classical complement cascade. IgM does not require high concentrations of antibody, because each molecule of IgM has multiple C1q-binding sites. C4d is very often detected in ABO-incompatible (ABOi) allografts without other evidence of rejection or graft dysfunction (discussed later in Sect. 1.3.4), and thus C4d alone is not a reliable indicator of HLA antibody-mediated graft injury or complement-induced damage. In addition, C4d is a possible product of both the classical (antibody-initiated) pathway and the lectin pathway, which also acts through C4. In contrast, the alternative pathway bypasses C4, as it relies on spontaneous C3 cleavage and C3b deposition on microbial surfaces. One report showed evidence for lectin pathway activation in C4d-positive renal allografts, based on simultaneous detection of the lectin pathway–specific molecule H-ficolin, suggesting that C4d might not be specific for antibody-dependent classical pathway activation in this setting [11].

Finally, experimental evidence indicates that HLA antibodies cause graft injury by additional complement-independent mechanisms. Indeed, the diagnostic criteria for AMR in renal and cardiac transplantation have recently been expanded to include recognition of C4d-negative AMR, based on clinical observations and molecular diagnostic studies showing AMR mechanisms involving endothelial injury and dysfunction in the absence of C4d deposition.

1.2.3.3 Why Might C4d Have Variable Organ-Specific Clinical Utility?

Local production of complement proteins by different organs may reduce the specificity of C4d in the diagnosis of AMR. Complement proteins are primarily synthesized by hepatocytes in the liver but are also produced locally by circulating monocytes, endothelial cells, resident macrophages, and gut epithelial cells. Many studies have demonstrated nonspecific C4d deposition, especially in the setting of tissue injury or due to local production of complement components, especially in liver allografts. In addition, C4d staining has been found to be variable and nonspecific for AMR in the lung, where C3d and C4d were found during infection [12–14]. Moreover, C4d is observed in the lamina propria and submucosal arterial branches of healthy bowel, and therefore, the clinical utility of C4d for diagnosis of small bowel transplant rejection is uncertain [15].

In conclusion, C4d is a cleavage product of both the classical and the lectin complement pathways, which remains covalently linked to proteins on the cell membrane at the site of complement activation. Its immunohistological detection in the microvasculature of renal, cardiac, and pancreas allografts is important, but not indispensable, for the diagnosis of HLA AMR. However, its utility in other solid organs, including lung, liver, and small bowel allografts, remains unreliable.

1.2.4 Crossmatching

Throughout the years, transplantation of patients with DSAs to potential allografts has been avoided through the use of a cell-based crossmatch test that employs patient serum and donor lymphocytes to determine whether or not there are circulating antidonor antibodies. The donor-specific crossmatch has evolved from complement-dependent cytotoxicity methods developed in the 1970s, with increasing sensitivity owing to anti-human globulin (AHG) augmentation and now to flow-cytometry-based methods developed in the 1980s (Fig. 1.8). Kidney transplant recipients are crossmatched with their potential donors pre-transplant, whereas crossmatching for recipients of heart and lung transplants occur perioperatively. Following implementation of the crossmatch test, the incidence of hyperacute rejection was vastly reduced. The original complement-dependent microlymphocytotoxicity crossmatch test has undergone several modifications to increase its sensitivity and reduce false-positive reactions by extending incubation times, treating serum to disrupt IgM antibodies, adding anti–human globulin reagents to enhance complement fixation and modifying wash steps to reduce background killing. Introduction of the flow cytometry crossmatch test in the 1980s (Fig. 1.8) significantly increased the sensitivity of the lymphocyte crossmatch test and also provided a measurement of both complement-fixing and non–complement-fixing HLA antibodies.

The introduction of solid-phase (i.e., cell-free) antibody testing platforms has improved both sensitivity and specificity of HLA and non-HLA antibody identification, even in broadly reactive sera. These new methods have made "virtual" crossmatches possible for most patients [16]. The virtual crossmatch compares the antibody specificities present in the recipient's serum with the donor's HLA type to assess crossmatch compatibility prior to transplant (Fig. 1.9). The ability to perform the virtual crossmatch is dependent on recent HLA antibody testing on the recipient and donor HLA typing that is inclusive of all antigens to which the patient has antibodies. The Organ Procurement and Transplantation Network (OPTN) has established a mechanism to enter "unacceptable" HLA for transplant candidates based on antibody identification using solid-phase tests, which are used to virtually cross-match donors for organ allocation in the United States. The virtual crossmatch has improved allocation of deceased donor kidneys by reducing offers to sensitized patients with known DSAs and who previously would have undergone time-consuming physical crossmatch testing before declining the offer.

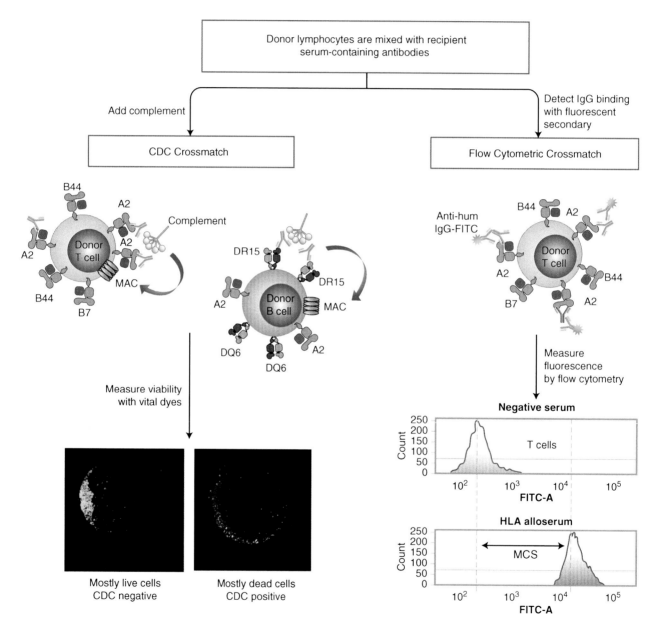

Fig. 1.8 Cell-based crossmatching. (*Left*), The complement-dependent lymphocytotoxicity assay tests the capacity of the transplant recipient's serum to kill donor T and B lymphocytes in the presence of complement. Dead lymphocytes (*red fluorescence*) are discriminated from live lymphocytes (CFDA; *green fluorescence*) by incorporation of a vital dye (propidium iodide) and scored as negative 1 (<20 %), 2 (20–40 %), 4 (40–60 %), 6 (60–80 %), or 8 (>80 %) killing. A score of 4 or greater is considered positive. (*Right*), Binding of recipient anti–HLA antibodies to donor T cells labeled with anti-CD3 PE and B cells labeled with anti-CD19 PE mAbs are detected by a fluorescent secondary anti–human Fitc–conjugated anti–human IgG F(ab')2 antibody. The amount of antibody bound to the cell corresponds to the fluorescence intensity, which is determined using a flow cytometer. The amount of anti–human IgG antibody bound to lymphocytes treated with normal human control IgG (MFI) is subtracted from the MFI of the recipient serum to determine the result. A score of greater than 50 MCS for the T-cell flow crossmatch and greater than 100 MCS for the B-cell flow crossmatch is considered positive

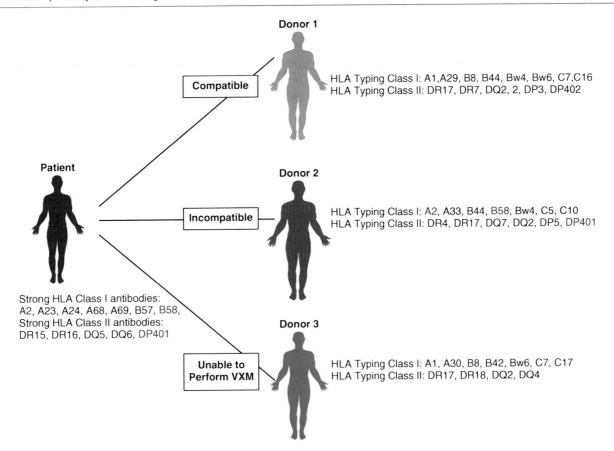

Fig. 1.9 Virtual crossmatch prediction. Virtual crossmatching requires recent antibody testing of the patient's sera by solid-phase flow and/or Luminex single-antigen bead arrays and complete HLA typing of the donor. In the example, the patient displays only strong antibodies to the specificities that are shown. A virtual crossmatch between the patient and Donor 1 indicates that the pair would be compatible because the patient does not display any DSA to this donor. The patient and Donor 2 are incompatible because the patient displays 3 strong DSA to this donor (A2, B58, DP401—highlighted in *red*). A virtual crossmatch cannot be performed for Donor 3 because the donor's HLA typing at the DP locus is lacking

1.2.5 Measuring Sensitization to HLA

The development of multiplex-bead arrays facilitated parallel testing of multiple-target HLA in a single reaction. Three common formats of solid-phase tests for anti-HLA antibodies are in use today. Screening tests for anti-HLA antibody include class I and class II HLA purified separately from several individuals that cover a broad spectrum of HLA antigens. These tests provide a positive or negative result but do not yield information on the specificity of the antibody. Panel-reactive antibody (PRA) tests have an HLA class I or class II phenotype from one individual attached to each bead. These tests provide a percent PRA result (the percentage of positive reactions) and can be used to assign antibody specificity depending on the breadth of antibodies present in the serum. The single HLA antigen tests have individual HLA antigens produced by recombinant DNA technologies attached to each bead (Fig. 1.10). These tests provide precise identification of individual antibody specificities and a relative measure of the amount of antibody present indicated by the mean fluorescent intensity (MFI).

> **Box 1.4**
>
> Most immunogenetics laboratories have attempted to define thresholds for assessing the clinical risk for a particular antibody by correlating the strength of the solid-phase test result with the crossmatch test. A major clinical question that remains to be answered is the risk of weak antibodies detected in these sensitive solid-phase assays. Clearly, there is considerable variability among transplant programs in the risk they assign to weak antibodies. This is not surprising, and in fact would be expected, based on the transplant program's risk tolerance, size and experience with transplants with a risk of antibody-mediated rejection, the patient's immunological history, and tolerance for aggressive treatment or donor characteristics. Efforts to develop standards for interpreting solid-phase test results should reduce variability in the future.

There are several limitations in the solid-phase assays that deserve mention. The different test formats present antigens at differing densities, and within each test format, there may be variable densities of HLA coupled to each bead and variation within different lots of beads. High antigen densities may distort antibody avidity so that very weak antibodies are detected that would not bind effectively to antigen present at a much lower density on a cell. Antibodies that react with epitopes that are shared by many different HLA such as Bw4 or Bw6, may not bind with the same apparent strength as those directed against epitopes that are unique to one antigen. Despite these limitations, there is strong evidence that there is a relationship between the amount of antibody detected in solid-phase tests and clinical outcomes and that most of the controversy centers on the role of weak antibodies. The MFI readout of the assay is intended to be a qualitative metric. Clinically, although higher MFIs correlate with increased binding of anti-HLA antibodies in the flow crossmatch and worse outcomes, there is still a wide range of MFI over which clinical consequences are not clearly defined. Single HLA–antigen bead assays have been modified to distinguish complement-fixing antibodies from non–complement-fixing using C1q and C3d detection reagents. Although HLA antibodies that fix complement are associated with higher rates of rejection and allograft loss, non–complement-binding antibodies still have documented clinical consequences.

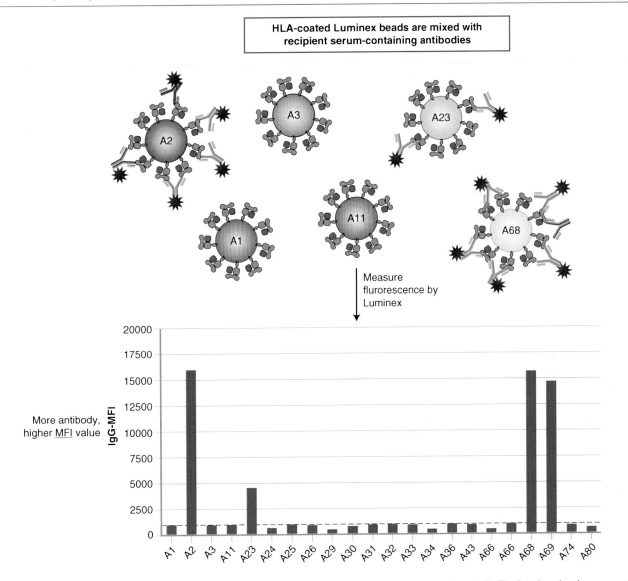

Fig. 1.10 Solid-phase Luminex detection of HLA antibodies. The Luminex bead-based antibody identification technology consists of a series of 100 polystyrene beads (subset shown) with single HLA molecules attached. Each bead is internally labeled with different ratios of two red fluorochromes, giving each bead a unique signal. The patient's serum is mixed with the single-antigen bead mix and the binding of anti–HLA antibodies is detected using a secondary PE-labeled anti–human IgG antibody (*red asterisk*). The Luminex beads are passed through two lasers in a single profile. One laser excites the red fluorochrome in the beads, while the other excites the PE bound to the second antibody. Emitted light from excited PE molecules is detected and expressed as MFI, which corresponds to the strength of the HLA antibody. The histogram shows antibody binding to A2 and A68 antigens at ~15,000 MFI and to A23 at ~5000 MFI

1.2.6 Pre-transplant HLA Antibody Assessment

A patient's sensitization status is a reflection of his or her exposure to allogenic stimuli including pregnancy, previous transplant, and transfusions. Furthermore, other immune stimuli such as infections and vaccinations can increase sensitization to HLA. Renal transplant candidates are typically monitored for changes in allosensitization on a quarterly basis and within 2–4 weeks of a sensitizing event. In the United States, highly sensitized patients have access to deceased donor kidneys nationwide and receive additional waitlist points for predicted virtual crossmatch-compatible deceased donor kidneys. Highly sensitized patients may undergo desensitization therapy using B-cell depletion, antibody removal, and immunomodulatory therapies. The efficacy of the desensitization therapy can be monitored using solid-phase phenotyping or single-antigen beads.

> **Box 1.5**
> Kidney paired donation (KPD) has become a powerful approach for facilitating living-donor transplantation for blood group– and HLA-allosensitized incompatible donor/recipient pairs. Incompatible donors, in essence, are exchanged to a compatible recipient. KPD has the capacity to achieve a completely negative crossmatch for the recipient, with no detectable DSA or blood type incompatibility. Finding such matches remains extraordinarily difficult for patients who are broadly sensitized and it is not always possible to find a donor with a completely negative crossmatch. In this situation, KPD may be coupled with desensitization therapy to lower the risk of AMR.

There is increasing evidence that up-to-date antibody profiles are important for the life-saving organs (heart, lung, liver, bowel) as well. Heart patients with mechanical-assist devices need blood and platelet support and, as a result, are prone to sensitization that may change frequently. With the improving accuracy of virtual crossmatches, the potential donor pool for the sensitized candidates for these organs can be geographically expanded, permitting shipping of organs recovered at distant hospitals and improving the chances for a compatible organ.

1.2.7 Post-transplant HLA Antibody Assessment

Growing evidence supports the role of HLA antibodies in acute and chronic allograft rejection, underscoring the need to detect these antibodies in a clinically relevant manner. The development of anti-HLA antibodies following transplantation is also positively associated with chronic rejection of heart, renal, lung, and liver allografts. Thus, post-transplant assessment of HLA antibodies may be useful in identifying patients at risk for acute and/or chronic rejection. The frequency of rejection episodes and production of anti–donor HLA antibodies has been found to be associated with an increased risk of developing transplant vasculopathy, which is a major manifestation of chronic rejection. When renal transplant patients were examined prospectively for the development of anti-HLA antibodies, there was a strong association between the production of DSAs, AMR, and early graft dysfunction. In addition, in a multicenter large-scale prospective study, the presence of HLA antibodies was confirmed in patients with well-functioning grafts; this detection predicted later graft failure. These studies demonstrate that assessment of DSA production after transplantation may identify patients at risk for AMR, early graft dysfunction, and/or the development of chronic rejection [17]. The utilization of post-transplant antibody assessment to identify patients at risk for acute and chronic rejection is appealing because it provides a means to monitor the patient in a less-invasive manner than surveillance biopsy; it is less expensive and can be repeated often.

> **Box 1.6**
> A major question is what therapeutic strategy should be employed once a patient tests positive for post-transplant anti–donor antibodies. It has been recommended that to treat and prevent AMR, APCs should be inhibited or depleted. Clinical trials are under way to investigate the efficacy of plasmapheresis combined with B depletional agents such as rituximab or the proteosome inhibitor bortezomib that targets metabolically active plasma cells. More research is needed to develop and investigate the application of novel therapies to prevent antibody synthesis and treat AMR.

1.2.8 Mechanisms of Graft Damage by HLA Antibodies

A key feature of chronic rejection is transplant vasculopathy, which is characterized by intimal proliferation of allograft blood vessels. Studies from our group and others have demonstrated that the signaling events elicited by crosslinking HLA molecules with antibodies stimulates proliferation of endothelial cells and smooth muscle cells, contributing to the process of transplant vasculopathy. We have shown that, because HLA classes I and II do not have intrinsic kinase activity, they must partner with other proteins that have the capacity to transduce intracellular signals. Ligation of HLA class I with antibodies increases association with integrin β4, which in turn, activates the intracellular signal cascade [18]. Integrin β4 is an important cell adhesion protein regulating cell adhesion, proliferation, migration, and survival. Blockade of integrin β4 impairs HLA antibody–stimulated signal transduction. Protein(s) that partner with HLA class II to transduce signaling are not yet known. However, ligation of either HLA class I or class II with antibodies activates mammalian target of rapamycin (mTOR) signaling through the SRC/FAK-PI3K-AKT pathway. mTOR is a central regulator of cell survival, proliferation and migration. mTOR exists in two distinct molecular complexes: mTOR complex 1 (mTORC1) composed of mTOR, GβL, and Raptor; and mTOR complex 2 (mTORC2) composed of mTORC2, GβL, Rictor, and Sin1 (Fig. 1.11).

The degree of HLA molecular aggregation stimulated by antibodies determines which complex is preferentially activated. We showed that ligation of HLA I molecules with low titer antibodies predominantly activates the mTORC2 pathway and upregulates cell survival proteins on the endothelium including Bcl-2 and Bcl-xL. Pretreatment of low titer of HLA class I antibodies protects the endothelium from cytotoxic T cell–mediated and complement-mediated injury in a mouse model. However, we posit that long-term exposure of the endothelium to low levels of HLA I antibodies will ultimately result in activation of complement or recruitment of monocytes, which in turn, may cause graft injury. Conversely, ligation of HLA I molecules with high titer of antibodies stimulates intracellular signals that promote endothelial cell proliferation via mTORC1. mTORC1 activates p70 ribosomal protein S6 kinase (S6K), which then phosphorylates S6 ribosomal protein (S6RP) and 4E-BP1 proteins. S6RP is required for protein synthesis and cell proliferation. We have demonstrated that phosphorylation of S6RP in endothelial cells in vitro is increased in response to treatment with HLA class I or class II antibodies. These in vitro findings are confirmed by in vivo studies using a murine heart allograft model in which phosphorylation of these proteins is increased in the endothelium of mice treated with MHC-I antibody, and in cardiac allograft biopsies undergoing AMR. Sirolimus (rapamycin) and its analog everolimus (U.S. Food and Drug Administration [FDA]–approved immunosuppressive agents for solid organ transplant) inhibit mTORC1 signaling at lower concentration, whereas both mTORC1 and mTORC2 signaling are inhibited by prolonged treatment or high concentration of rapamycin. Our group has shown that treatment with rapamycin or everolimus blocks HLA class I antibody–induced phosphorylation of S6K and S6RP and proliferation in endothelial cells and, therefore, may be an effective therapy to prevent transplant vasculopathy [19].

Therefore, we hypothesize that phosphorylated S6RP or phosphorylated S6K may be predictive of clinical response to rapamycin treatment; that is, patients with high level of phosphorylated S6RP or phosphorylated S6K on the biopsy would respond better to sirolimus treatment than those with low expression. Consistent with our hypothesis, the high level of phosphorylated S6RP in metastatic sarcomas is correlated with early clinical response to mTOR inhibitor treatment [20].

Fig. 1.11 Intracellular signaling activated by HLA antibodies. Treatment of endothelial cells with HLA class I or class II antibodies activates mTORC1, which in turn, increases phosphorylation of S6K followed by S6RP and 4E-BP1. Ligation of HLA class I molecules with low-titer antibodies prefers to activate the mTORC2 pathway and upregulates cell survival proteins on the endothelium including Bcl-2 and Bcl-xL. Rapamycin can block activation of mTORC1 or mTORC2 upon higher concentration or extended time

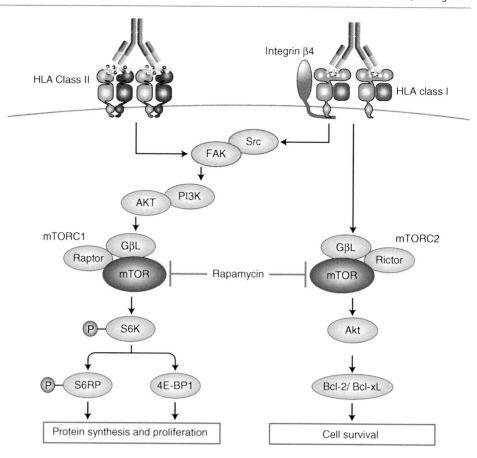

1.3 The Role of Non-HLA in Organ Transplantation

1.3.1 Clinical Importance of Non–HLA Antibodies in Organ Transplantation

Currently, more and more evidence has shown that non-HLA antibodies contribute to the pathogenesis of acute and chronic rejection and decreased long-term graft survival of solid organ transplants [21]. The clinical relevance of non-HLA antibodies has been demonstrated in the setting of 3100 HLA-identical sibling transplantations performed by Opelz et al [22]. The 10-year graft survival was 72.4 % for patients without HLA antibodies compared with 55.5 % for patients with HLA antibodies who had more than 50 % PRA. Although many of these non-HLA antibodies remain poorly defined, the principle antigenic targets are expressed on cells of the allograft including endothelium and epithelium. The endothelium constitutes the inner cellular lining of the blood vessels and the lymphatic system. Therefore, donor endothelial cells are in direct contact with the recipient's circulating peripheral blood lymphocytes and have been shown to be the major immunological targets for the pathogenesis of allograft rejection. The non-HLA antibodies can be classified as either alloantigens, such as the MHC class I chain–related gene A (MICA) or MICB, or tissue-specific autoantigens such as vimentin, cardiac myosin (CM), collagen V (Col V), agrin, and angiotensin II receptor type I (AT1R).

1.3.1.1 MICA Antibodies

MICA is a highly polymorphic gene located in the HLA class I region between HLA class I and HLA class II genes, with 100 alleles described. The MICA gene contains a heat shock response element (HRE) promoter and its expression level can be induced in response to cellular stress, but MICA mRNA levels are not affected by inflammatory cytokines such as interferon-γ (IFN-γ), unlike HLA. MICA antigens act as ligands of the activating NKG2D receptor on NK cells, on γ/δ subgroups of T lymphocytes, and on α/β subgroups of CD8+ T lymphocytes. In contrast to classical HLA, MICA does not bind β2-microglobulin or exhibit conventional class I peptide binding.

Alloantibodies against MICA have been found to be associated with acute and chronic vascular rejection in renal and heart transplantation. Presensitization to MICA causes acute rejection and decreases long-term graft survival. MICA antibodies have been found to cause CDC against endothelial cells from the graft, suggesting these antibodies can cause complement-mediated damage of the donor endothelium.

1.3.1.2 Autoantibodies

Under normal circumstances, vimentin, K-α1 tubulin, CM, and Col V are not expressed on the cell surface. During trans-plantation, the cold ischemia-reperfusion injury (IRI) and the alloimmune responses through direct and indirect pathways cause initial damage to the graft. In this setting, the intracellular self-antigens can be translocated to the cell surface during apoptosis or released during necrosis. High-affinity antibody production by B cells to a particular target is dependent on sufficient help from antigen-specific T cells. Studies have shown that that repetitive exposure of autoantigens at higher frequency breaks anergy of autoreactive T cells. These antigens can also be presented via the indirect recognition pathway to generate pathogenic allo- and autoreactive cellular and antibody-mediated immune responses. The indirect pathway involves processing of the donor alloantigens and/or self-antigens by recipient APCs and presentation to recipient T cells and is believed to be the major pathway for chronic rejection. Anti-vimentin antibodies, anti-K-α1 tubulin antibodies, anti-Col V, and anti-AT1R-antibodies have all been demonstrated in chronic rejection.

The indirect alloimmune response, once initiated, can spread to additional determinants within the primary target antigen, called intramolecular epitope spreading. Through these mechanisms, the development of antibody-mediated responses to autoantigens could result as a consequence of alloimmune-mediated graft damage where repeated exposure of recipient CD4+ T cells to self-antigens surpasses the threshold of self-tolerance and leads to autoimmunity. In addition, repeated stimulation of CD4+ T cells with self-antigens can lead to the development of autoantibody-inducing CD4+ T cells. Therefore, chronic stimulation with autoantigens can break T-cell self-tolerance. Administration of anti-MHC class I antibodies into the native lungs of mice showed increased expression of interleukin-17 (IL-17) and subsequent development of antibodies to self-antigens K-α1 tubulin and Col V [23]. Thus, during transplantation, autoimmunity can result from overstimulating the host's immune response by repeated immunization with antigens.

1.3.2 Graft Damage Caused by Non-HLA Antibodies

Non-HLA antibodies cause graft damage through both complement-dependent and -independent pathways [24]. Complement-fixing IgG or IgM antibody bind to these antigens on the surface of vascular endothelium and can potentially interact with C1q to activate the classical complement cascade, resulting in damage to the target graft. In addition, studies of different animal IRI models showed that reperfusion of ischemic tissues elicits an acute inflammatory response involving the complement system, which is activated by autoreactive natural IgM [25]. Non-HLA antibodies such as anti-MICA antibodies and anti-vimentin antibodies have all been found to mediate CDC in vitro, suggesting that they may contribute to the pathogenesis of AMR through complement-mediated injury.

Anti-K-α1 tubulin antibodies, anti-vimentin antibodies, and AT1R-antibodies have been shown to cause graft injury through complement-independent pathways [24–27]. These antibodies transduce proinflammatory and proliferative signals, suggesting a mechanistic role in both acute and chronic allograft rejection. Anti-vimentin antibodies have been shown to induce the expression of P-selectin on the microvessels of hearts.

Anti-vimentin antibodies may also indirectly trigger endothelial cell (EC) activation by stimulating leukocytes to release platelet-activating factor and subsequent platelet activation and adherence to the endothelium. The binding of K-α1 tubulin antibodies to airway epithelial cells activates a protein kinase C (PKC)–driven calcium maintenance pathway and stimulates expression of transcription factors and fibrogenic growth factors, culminating in cell cycle signaling and fibroproliferation [24].

AT1R Ab has been demonstrated to induce severe vasoconstriction in arteries of the renal allograft but not in native arteries in a kidney transplant animal model. Interestingly, the vasoconstriction caused by AT1R Ab is significantly stronger and longer than vasoconstriction caused by angiotensin II under normal physiological circumstances. AT1R Ab has also been demonstrated to induce upregulation of tissue factor in human monocytes and the angiotensin-converting enzyme (ACE) inhibitor, losartan, significantly inhibited tissue factor induced by angiotensin II vitro. AT1R-Abs induced vasoconstriction, upregulation of tissue factor, along with an increase in AT1R expression induced by ischemic injury during transplantation can trigger artery thrombosis. Dragun et al [26] demonstrated that AT1R Ab caused small artery thrombosis and positive tissue factor staining on renal biopsies in patients with AMR, and the risk of graft failure is significantly higher in renal transplant recipients with AT1R Ab, particularly when concurrent with HLA DSA [27].

1.3.3 Assessment of Non-HLA Antibodies Before and After Transplantation

In the past, the importance of anti–endothelial cell antibodies (AECA, or non–HLA antibodies) in allograft rejection has been underestimated. Currently, the routine lymphocyte crossmatching techniques fail to detect AECAs. Non–HLA endothelial cell antibodies can be detected by endothelial cell crossmatching. Antibodies to MICA or AT1R are detected by solid-phase assays employing Luminex technology and enzyme-linked immunosorbent assay (ELISA), respectively. The XM-One assay is another novel endothelial cell flow cytometry crossmatch technique that uses Tie-2 antibody–coated magnetic beads to select precursor EC directly from donor blood, and these cells are reacted with patient serum to identify AECAs (Fig. 1.12). Results of a multicenter clinical trial evaluating the association of AECAs with renal allograft rejection showed that pretransplant donor-reactive AECAs were present in a significantly higher proportion of patients with rejection [28]. Additional studies are needed to confirm if this crossmatch method is useful for identifying clinically relevant AECAs.

A major limitation of current studies is the lack of knowledge of the antigenic specificity of these AECAs. Because AECAs can be detected in a wide variety of clinical pathologies that involve the vascular system, such as systemic lupus erythematosus (SLE), rheumatoid arthritis (RA), and vasculitides, it is important to distinguish de novo autoantibodies from the recurrence of the original disease. In addition, it is also critical to establish a pre-transplant base level of non–HLA antibodies to understand the relevance of these antibodies to graft rejection.

Continued efforts to define the non–HLA alloantigens and tissue-specific autoantigens involved in transplant rejection are essential for understanding the mechanisms and pathogenesis of non–HLA antibodies and development of treatment options.

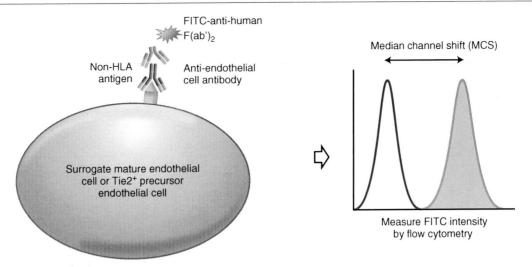

Fig. 1.12 Endothelial cell crossmatching. The patient's serum is incubated with endothelial cells. If the serum displays antibodies against antigens expressed on endothelial cells, these antibodies will bind to endothelial cells. The amount of AECAs bound to the cell corresponds to the fluorescence intensity, which is determined using a flow cytometer. The amount of anti–human IgG antibody bound to lymphocytes treated with normal human control IgG (MFI) is subtracted from the MFI of the patient's serum to determine the result

1.3.4 ABOi Transplantation

ABO blood group antigens are glycoproteins present on red blood cells and vascular endothelium. ABO antibodies develop naturally after gut colonization with *Escherichia coli*, typically at about 6–8 months of age. Without preconditioning to lower the level of circulating ABO antibodies, the recipient's preformed natural antibodies react with A and/or B carbohydrate antigens expressed on the vascular endothelial cells in the ABOi graft: antibody binding leads to complement fixation and activation; downstream endothelial cell activation and damage cause the formation of microthrombi and microhemorrhages, resulting in hyperacute rejection within minutes.

With the increasing need of donors for solid organ transplantation, various efforts have been made to enlarge the donor pool, including increasing acceptance of deceased donor grafts with marginal quality, developing paired exchange programs for live kidney transplantation, and establishing desensitization protocols for patients with preformed HLA antibodies or patients with incompatible ABO blood groups. Nowadays, successful ABOi transplants can be achieved by pre-transplant reduction of ABO blood group antibodies through repeated plasmapheresis combined with B-cell depletion and the use of IVIG. Although an anti-ABO level below a serological titer of approximately 1:16 is sufficient for successful ABOi transplants, most centers aim to achieve titers of 1:8 or less. In children younger than 2 years, ABOi transplants have been quite successful because antibody production is not yet fully developed in infants [28]. In addition, there is also a developmental lag in T-cell responses to ABO antigens. Currently, infants younger than 24 months listed for ABOi heart transplants with the United Network for Organ Sharing (UNOS) are required to have titer assays run when listed and are checked monthly until a heart becomes available. When an organ offer is accepted, a confirmatory titer test is run immediately before proceeding with donor arrangements. UNOS policy requires an ABO titer of 1:4 or less to proceed with transplantation. The outstanding ABOi transplant results are due not only to effective desensitization protocols but also to routine post-transplant surveillance, early detection, and an enhanced therapeutic approach for AMR.

ABOi living-donor kidney transplantation has been routinely performed in Japan since 1989 owing to the limited organ supply in this country. The long-term patient survival has been found to be comparable between ABOi recipients and ABO-compatible (ABOc) matched controls in two recent studies from both Japan [29] and the United States [30]. However, the cumulative incidence of graft loss was higher among ABOi recipients than that observed in ABOc recipients in the U.S. cohort. This difference was attributed only to an increased rate of graft loss during the first 14 days

after transplantation. A recent study showed a significantly higher incidence of early death from infection in ABOi recipients during the first post-transplant year. Plasmapheresis is the most common method used to remove antibodies. This procedure eliminates approximately 20 % of preformed anti-ABO antibodies with each session. However, this technique also removes coagulation factors, hormones, and antiviral and antibacterial antibodies, therefore increasing the risk of bleeding and infection. It has also been suggested that infection in ABOi recipients can result in neutralizing antibodies that are cross-reactive with mismatched ABO blood group antigens expressed on the surface of allograft vascular endothelium, sometimes causing acute AMR that leads to organ failure or loss.

ABOi heart transplantation is increasing in the pediatric population. Following an initial report by West et al [31], several transplant networks are now allowing ABOi listing for pediatric heart candidates. Analysis of the Pediatric Heart Transplant Study database of patients younger than 15 months revealed reduced rejection and no differences in mortality in 85 ABOi cardiac transplants compared with 502 ABOc recipients transplanted between 1996 and 2008 [28]. However, ABOi heart transplantation in adults has not been as successful. The incidence of death or retransplantation in the ABOi recipients was twice as high as the ABOc group at both 30 days and 1 year after transplant from an International Society for Heart & Lung Transplantation (ISHLT) registry study of 76,663 adult heart recipients transplanted between 1988 and 2011 [31]. ABOi grafts surviving past the first year after transplant, however, had a similar incidence of failure compared with the ABOc group. However, the incidence of death or retransplantation in the most recent cohort of recipients transplanted across the ABO barrier after 2005 appears to have similar short-term and long-term outcomes compared with that in ABOc transplantation [31]. These results indicate an ABOi heart transplant may be an option for carefully selected adult patients with advanced heart disease who otherwise would not have an organ available.

Interestingly, anti–ABO blood group antibodies may return to high levels after the transplant without causing apparent damage to the graft. Alexandre et al [32] first described this phenomenon, called "accommodation," in recipients of deliberate ABOi kidneys. The mechanism underlying graft accommodation remains unclear. Platt et al [33] proposed three possible mechanisms for this phenomenon, postulating that either the antibody or the antigen was somehow modulated in the graft or, alternatively, that the graft itself became resistant to the damaging effects of antibodies. There is some evidence now to support the latter possibility—that cells exposed to low levels of antibody may express antiapoptotic genes early after exposure; in the accommodated graft, a distinct phenotype characterized by expression of tumor necrosis factor-α (TNF-α), transforming growth factor-β1 (TGF-β1), SMAD5, protein kinase GFRA1, and MUC1 is observed 3 months or more following successful transplantation.

C4d deposition along peritubular capillaries is a hallmark for antibody-dependent complement activation. In ABOi transplants, C4d deposition in the absence of histological evidence of rejection is a common finding. C4d positivity is found in 94 % of ABOi kidney recipients on protocol biopsy compared with 11 % in ABOc patients. Further studies indicated that a lack of C4d staining correlated with graft failure due to chronic rejection events, indicating that C4d deposition may be a favorable prognostic factor in this group of patients [34].

In conclusion, the dogma that ABO blood group incompatibility should be considered an absolute contraindication to kidney transplantation has been challenged over the past two decades. Various efforts have been made to establish standardized protocols, and recent advances in the treatment of AMRs have led to excellent graft survival rates equivalent to those of ABOc transplants in selected kidney and pediatric heart recipients.

1.4 Case Studies

1.4.1 Case Study 1. HLA Typing by Molecular Methods Results in Improved Accuracy Over Serological Methods

The patient is a 46-year-old African American woman with a history of end-stage renal disease, stemming from hypoplastic kidneys. The patient initially underwent a living related renal transplant from her father (Donor #1) in 1983. At that time, the patient, her mother and father, and two siblings were HLA-typed by serological methods (Table 1.1). The kidney lasted approximately 13 years, at which time, the patient again started dialysis and was relisted for a deceased-donor kidney. After 6 years, the patient received her second transplant (Donor #2) in 2001 from a deceased donor. This kidney lasted for approximately 12 years. HLA typing on the patient, now being evaluated for a third transplant, was repeated using molecular methods in 2013, and the typing results were found to be discrepant from the typing performed in 1983. The serological typing initially performed in 1983 identified only one antigen at the HLA A locus on the patient, father, mother, and both brothers. Retyping of the patient using molecular methods showed that the patient is heterozygous at the HLA A locus and carries A2 and A74.

Furthermore, the patient's initial serological typing at class II was low resolution and was reported at the level of broad groups, DR2, 8 and DQ1, 3, whereas the more recent higher-resolution molecular typing was determined to be DR12, 15 and DQ5, 6. The broad group antigens DR2 and DQ1 are represented in the newer results by the higher-resolution DR15 and DQ6, respectively. However, the broad group antigens DR8 and DQ3 were not confirmed in the more recent typing, and we conclude that one haplotype was initially reported incorrectly in 1983.

Table 1.1 HLA typing of patient, donor, and family

Year	Typing method		A	B	HLA		DQ
					DRB1	DRB345	
1983	Serology	Patient	2	35	2		1
			X	42	8		3
		Donor #1, father	2	35	2		1
			X	5	7		X
		Mother	30	5			
			X	42			
		Brother #1	2	5			
			X	42			
		Brother #2	2	35			
			X	42			
2001	Molecular, SSP	Donor #2, DD	2	39	4	53	8
			24	51	14	52	7
2013	Molecular, SSO	Patient	2	35	15	51	6
			74	42	12	52	5

DD deceased donor, *X* presence of a second antigen is not identified.

1.4.2 Case Study 2. An Example of Early AMR Due to Production of DSA During Post-transplant Anamnestic Response

The patient is a 41-year-old Hispanic woman with a history of end-stage renal disease due to diabetes mellitus. The patient has had one known pregnancy, and no other known sensitizing events. The specificity and strength of HLA antibodies was first assessed in the patient's September 2007 (pre-transplant day –2618) sera sample by single-antigen bead assay. The patient was positive for antibodies to HLA class I antigens, and negative for antibodies to HLA class II antigens, with a cPRA of 92 % for all antibodies (Table 1.2). The patient was listed for a deceased-donor kidney/pancreas transplant in November 2008. Over time, the strength and specificities of the patient's antibodies fluctuated; however, the cPRA for all antibodies was 31 % within 30 days of transplant.

A local deceased donor became available for this patient in November 2014. HLA typing of the patient and donor by molecular methods are:

Recipient: A29, 30, B7, 64, Bw6, DR17, 4, DR52, 53, DQ2, 8
Donor #1: A24, 68, B35, 39, Bw6, C1, 7, DR14, DR52, DQ7

The patient had a history of DSA to A24 (2423 MFI) and A68 (1414 MFI) that was last seen in her March 2012 sera (–952 days pre-transplant; Fig. 1.13). At peak strength, the preformed DSA to A24 was 11,872 MFI at –2618 days pre-transplant. However, the patient did not display any DSA at the time of transplant, and as predicted, the T and B cytotoxicity and flow crossmatch results were negative. The patient was transplanted with solumedrol and thymoglobulin induction.

A serum was sent for single-antigen bead based testing on postoperative day (POD) 4. A DSA to A24 (1525 MFI) was reported. Subsequent single-antigen testing on POD 11 showed that the patient displayed DSAs to A24 (10,235 MFI), A68 (5386 MFI), B35 (10,298 MFI), and B39 (10,304 MFI). A histogram displaying the strength of antibodies to HLA class I antigens in the single-antigen bead test on POD 13 is shown in Fig. 1.14. Biopsy results showed acute antibody-mediated changes with C4d staining of peritubular capillaries and glomerular thrombotic microangiopathy, consistent with acute/active AMR. The patient was treated beginning on POD 13 with plasmapheresis for 5 days and IVIG. Velcade was also administered on POD 13 with a plan for 3 additional doses over the next 2 weeks. The strength of the patient's antibodies significantly reduced throughout the course of therapy.

Table 1.2 Pre-transplant cPRA for all antibodies over time

Day pre-transplant	cPRA, %
–2618	92
–2151	64
–1736	31
–1341	38
–1123	89
–952	90
–765	31
–394	34
–30	31

Fig. 1.13 Case study 2. The patient displays DSA identified by single-antigen bead test in pre- and post-transplant sera. The peak of the post-transplant immune response, at POD 11, shows DSA to A24, A68, B35, and B39. Treatment began on POD 13 (*arrow*). By POD 83, the strengths of all DSA were below the positive cutoff of 1000 MFI (*dotted line*).

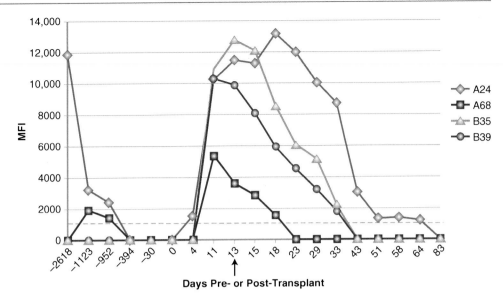

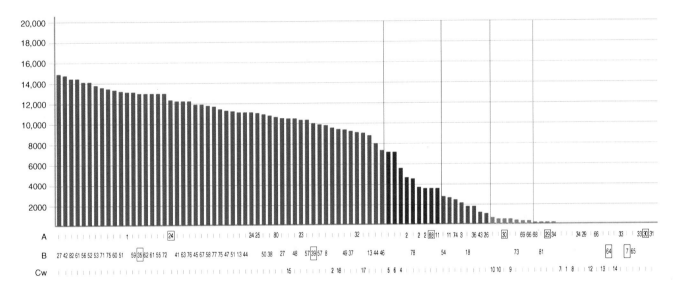

Fig. 1.14 Case study 2. Histogram shows reactivity to HLA class I single-antigen beads on POD 11. Each *bar*, representing one bead, indicates the strength of the antibody measured by MFI. HLA-A, -B, and -C specificities are shown. *Red boxes* indicate DSA. The patient also displays an abundance of antibodies to third-party antigens (i.e., those that are not donor-specific). Owing to self-tolerance, the patient does not display antibodies to self-antigens (*black boxes*)

1.4.3 Case Study 3. An Example of AMR Due to Nonadherence to Immunosuppressive Medication

The patient is a 20-year-old Hispanic woman with a history of end-stage renal disease secondary to renal hypoplasia. The patient received her first deceased-donor renal transplant in 2006 at age 12, but the graft failed secondary to medication noncompliance; hemodialysis was reinitiated in 2009. The patient was relisted, with a cPRA of 87 %.

In July 2012, a deceased donor became available. HLA typing of the patient and her first and second donors by molecular methods are:

Recipient: A24, 66, B39, 53, Bw6, DR4, 14, DR52, 53, DQ7, 8
Donor #1: A23, 24, B7, 35, Bw6, DR53, 51, DQ6, 3
Donor #2: A2, B39, 65, Bw6, Cw7, 8, DR4, 17, DQ52, 53, DQ2, 8, DQA1*03:01, 05:01, DPB1*02:01, 04:02

The patient did not have any preformed DSA to this donor, and as expected, the T and B CDC and flow cross-matches were negative. The patient was transplanted in July 2012. A de novo DSA to DQ2 (6847 MFI) was identified at routine single-antigen screening, approximately 2 years post-transplant, on POD 798. Approximately 1 month later, POD 827, the patient was biopsied owing to increasing creatinine and presence of DSA: A2 (2977 MFI), Cw8 (2377 MFI), and DQ2 (17,320) (Fig. 1.15). Biopsy results were positive for acute antibody-mediated changes with C4d staining of peritubular capillaries, consistent with acute/active AMR. Noncompliance to immunosuppressive medications was determined as a contributing factor for rejection. The patient was treated with plasmapheresis for 5 days and three doses of IVIG. The patient's creatinine improved, and was 3.2 as of POD 904 with good urine output. However, a single-antigen bead test indicates that the strength of the patient's DSA is increasing.

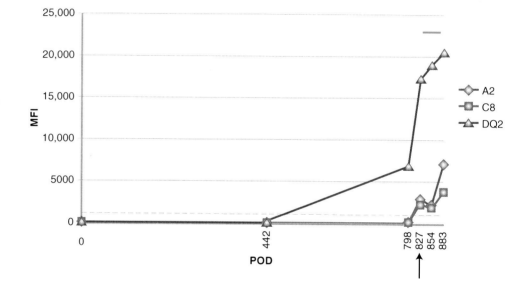

Fig. 1.15 Case study 3. DSA identified by a single-antigen bead test in post-transplant sera. *Dotted line* indicates positive cutoff of 1000 MFI. DSA to DQ2 was evident in the sera on POD 798. In the following sera, DSA to A2 and C8 were also present. The patient was treated with plasmapheresis and IVIG after POD 827 (*arrow*). Treatment dates are indicated by the *blue line*

1.4.4   Case Study 4. An Example of Acute Rejection and Vascular Changes in the Absence of HLA DSAs

The patient is a 46-year-old man with a history of end-stage renal disease secondary to possible glomerulonephritis. His first transplant was from a deceased donor in 1993 and functioned well until January 2007, when he resumed hemodialysis. The patient received a second deceased-donor transplant in February 2011.

HLA typing of the patient and his first and second donors by molecular methods are:

Recipient: A29, 66, B18, 44, Bw4, DR7, 15, DR51, 53, DQ2, 6
Donor #1: Unknown
Donor #2: A29, 31 B60, 44, Bw4, 6, Cw10, 16, DR7, DR53, DQ2, DQA1*02

Post-transplant, the patient was maintained on triple immune suppression and seen annually for routine clinic visits at our center; however, antibody screening was not performed until a sample was received in January 2015. The patient did not display any HLA DSAs. However, owing to rising creatinine, the patient was biopsied a week later and found to have acute cell-mediated rejection type IIA (vascular rejection) with mild interstitial fibrosis and tubular atrophy and concurrent peritubular capillary inflammation but was negative for C4d staining.

Because the biopsy was suggestive of AMR in the absence of HLA DSA, the presence of non–HLA antibodies was investigated in the same sera. The patient was negative for AECAs by the EC-XM on two surrogate endothelial cell lines. The patient was also negative for antibodies to MICA. However, the patient was positive for antibodies to AT1R at a level of greater than 40 U/mL (1:100 dilution; Fig. 1.16). The patient was treated with thymoglobulin and pulse steroids and started on an angiotensin receptor (AR) blocker. Plasmapheresis was also initiated and antibodies to AT1R were reduced to below the level of detection.

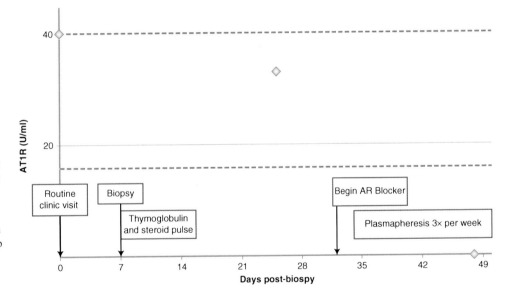

Fig. 1.16 Case study 4. AT1R antibody (*blue diamonds*) was measured in sera at a 1:100 dilution by AT1R ELSA on days 0, 26, and 48 and is expressed as U/mL. (Day 0 and day 26 sera were not tested for AT1R until the fifth week after the biopsy.) *Dotted lines* indicate the positive threshold at 17 U/mL and the top of the linear range, 40 U/mL. Treatment course is also displayed

References

1. Robinson J, Halliwell JA, Hayhurst JH, Flicek P, Parham P, Marsh SGE. The IPD and IMGT/HLA database: allele variant databases. Nucleic Acids Res. 2015;43(Database issue):D423–31.

2. Robinson J, Malik A, Parham P, Bodmer JG, Marsh SGE. IMGT/HLA: a sequence database for the human major histocompatibility complex. Tissue Antigens. 2000;55:280–7.

3. Takemoto SK, Terasaki PI, Gjertson DW, Cecka JM. Twelve years' experience with national sharing of HLA-matched cadaveric kidneys for transplantation. N Engl J Med. 2000;343:1078–84.

4. Afzali B, Lombardi G, Lechler RI. Pathways of major histocompatibility complex allorecognition. Curr Opin Organ Transplant. 2008; 13:438–44.

5. Angaswamy N, Tiriveedhi V, Sarma NJ, Subramanian V, Klein C, Wellen J, et al. Interplay between immune responses to HLA and non-HLA self-antigens in allograft rejection. Hum Immunol. 2013;74:1478–85.

6. Ridge JP, Di Rosa F, Matzinger P. A conditioned dendritic cell can be a temporal bridge between a CD4+ T-helper and a T-killer cell. Nature. 1998;393:474–8.

7. Thomas KA, Valenzuela MM, Reed EF. The perfect storm: HLA antibodies, complement, FcγRs, and endothelium in transplant rejection. Trends Mol Med. 2015;21:319–29.

8. Mathern DR, Heeger PS. Molecules great and small: the complement system. Clin J Am Soc Nephrol. 2015;10(9):1636-50.

9. González-Stawinski GV, Tan CD, Smedira NG, Starling RC, Rodríguez ER. Decay-accelerating factor expression may provide immunoprotection against antibody-mediated cardiac allograft rejection. J Heart Lung Transplant. 2008;27:357–61.

10. Tan CD, Sokos GG, Pidwell DJ, Smedira NG, Gonzalez-Stawinski GV, Taylor DO, et al. Correlation of donor-specific antibodies, complement and its regulators with graft dysfunction in cardiac antibody-mediated rejection. Am J Transplant. 2009;9:2075–84.

11. Imai N, Nishi S, Alchi B, Ueno M, Fukase S, Arakawa M, et al. Immunohistochemical evidence of activated lectin pathway in kidney allografts with peritubular capillary C4d deposition. Nephrol Dial Transplant. 2006;21:2589–95.

12. Roberts JA, Barrios R, Cagle PT, Ge Y, Takei H, Haque AK, et al. The presence of anti-HLA donor-specific antibodies in lung allograft recipients does not correlate with C4d immunofluorescence in transbronchial biopsy specimens. Arch Pathol Lab Med. 2014;138:1053–8.

13. Wallace WD, Reed EF, Ross D, Lassman CR, Fishbein MC. C4d staining of pulmonary allograft biopsies: an immunoperoxidase study. J Heart Lung Transplant. 2005;24:1565–70.

14. Westall GP, Snell GI, McLean C, Kotsimbos T, Williams T, Magro C. C3d and C4d deposition early after lung transplantation. J Heart Lung Transplant. 2008;27:722–8.

15. Troxell ML, Higgins JP, Kambham N. Evaluation of C4d staining in liver and small intestine allografts. Arch Pathol Lab Med. 2006;130:1489–96.

16. Baxter-Lowe LA, Cecka M, Kamoun M, Sinacore J, Melcher ML. Center-defined unacceptable HLA antigens facilitate transplants for sensitized patients in a multi-center kidney exchange program. Am J Transplant. 2014;14:1592–8.

17. Wiebe C, Gibson IW, Blydt-Hansen TD, Karpinski M, Ho J, Storsley LJ, et al. Evolution and clinical pathologic correlations of de novo donor-specific HLA antibody post kidney transplant. Am J Transplant. 2012;12:1157–67.

18. Zhang X, Rozengurt E, Reed EF. HLA class I molecules partner with integrin beta4 to stimulate endothelial cell proliferation and migration. Sci Signal. 2010;3:ra85.

19. Zhang X, Valenzuela NM, Reed EF. HLA class I antibody-mediated endothelial and smooth muscle cell activation. Curr Opin Organ Transplant. 2012;17:446–51.

20. Iwenofu OH, Lackman RD, Staddon AP, Goodwin DG, Haupt HM, Brooks JS. Phospho-S6 ribosomal protein: a potential new predictive sarcoma marker for targeted mTOR therapy. Mod Pathol. 2008;21:231–7.

21. Zhang Q, Reed EF. Non-MHC antigenic targets of the humoral immune response in transplantation. Curr Opin Immunol. 2010;22:682–8.

22. Opelz G. Collaborative Transplant Study. Non-HLA transplantation immunity revealed by lymphocytotoxic antibodies. Lancet. 2005;365:1570–6.

23. Braun RK, Molitor-Dart M, Wigfield C, Xiang Z, Fain SB, Jankowska-Gan E, et al. Transfer of tolerance to collagen type V suppresses T-helper-cell-17 lymphocyte-mediated acute lung transplant rejection. Transplantation. 2009;88:1341–8.

24. Dragun D, Catar R, Philippe A. Non-HLA antibodies in solid organ transplantation: recent concepts and clinical relevance. Curr Opin Organ Transplant. 2013;18:430–5.

25. Zhang M, Austen Jr WG, Chiu I, Alicot EM, Hung R, Ma M, et al. Identification of a specific self-reactive IgM antibody that initiates intestinal ischemia/reperfusion injury. Proc Natl Acad Sci U S A. 2004;101:3886–91.

26. Dragun D, Müller DN, Bräsen JH, Fritsche L, Nieminen-Kelhä M, Dechend R, et al. Angiotensin II type 1-receptor activating antibodies in renal-allograft rejection. N Engl J Med. 2005;352:558–69.

27. Taniguchi M, Rebellato LM, Cai J, Hopfield J, Briley KP, Haisch CE, et al. Higher risk of kidney graft failure in the presence of anti-angiotensin II type-1 receptor antibodies. Am J Transplant. 2013; 13:2577–89.

28. Henderson HT, Canter CE, Mahle WT, Dipchand AI, LaPorte K, Schechtman KB, et al. ABO-incompatible heart transplantation: analysis of the Pediatric Heart Transplant Study (PHTS) database. J Heart Lung Transplant. 2012;31:173–9.

29. Takahashi K, Saito K, Takahara S, Okuyama A, Tanabe K, Toma H, et al. Excellent long-term outcome of ABO-incompatible living donor kidney transplantation in Japan. Am J Transplant. 2004;4:1089–96.

30. Montgomery JR, Berger JC, Warren DS, James NT, Montgomery RA, Segev DL. Outcomes of ABO-incompatible kidney transplantation in the United States. Transplantation. 2012;93:603–9.

31. West LJ, Pollock-Barziv SM, Dipchand AI, Lee KJ, Cardella CJ, Benson LN, et al. ABO-incompatible heart transplantation in infants. N Engl J Med. 2001;344:793–800.

32. Alexandre GP, Squifflet JP, De Bruyère M, Latinne D, Reding R, Gianello P, et al. Present experiences in a series of 26 ABO-incompatible living donor renal allografts. Transplant Proc. 1987; 19:4538–42.

33. Platt JL, Cascalho M, West L. Lessons from cardiac transplantation in infancy. Pediatr Transplant. 2009;13:814–9.

34. Haas M, Segev DL, Racusen LC, Bagnasco SM, Locke JE, Warren DS, et al. C4d deposition without rejection correlates with reduced early scarring in ABO-incompatible renal allografts. JASN. 2009; 20:197–204.

Heart Transplant Pathology

Michael C. Fishbein

Heart transplantation has become standard therapy for patients with end-stage heart disease from a variety of causes. Whereas more noninvasive methods for detecting rejection are evolving, right ventricular endomyocardial biopsy remains the gold standard.

2.1 Technical Considerations (Fig. 2.1)

Evaluation of endomyocardial biopsies is performed on small samples of a large organ, typically from one region, the right side of the interventricular septum. If the free wall of the right ventricle is biopsied, that is unintentional owing to the risk of perforation. A total of four fragments of tissue sampled is generally regarded as adequate, but more is usually better. If the biopsy is composed of fewer than three fragments of myocardium, the biopsy should be considered suboptimal, and this fact should be reported. The biopsies may be fixed and processed routinely with multiple levels from each block evaluated. H&E staining is sufficient for most biopsies. Elastic and trichrome stains may help to distinguish endocardial from myocardial tissue. (See Appendix for UCLA biopsy protocols.) This distinction is important to distinguish Quilty lesions (QLs) from acute cell-mediated rejection (ACR). Fresh-frozen tissue can be utilized for immunofluorescence (IF) studies for the evaluation of antibody-mediated rejection (AMR). However, immunohistochemical (IHC) studies of paraffin-embedded tissue are also useful in this regard with only slight loss of sensitivity [1]. In some centers, all biopsies are frozen or rush same-day processing is utilized for rapid diagnosis. At UCLA, biopsies are processed overnight and read out the next morning; in our experience, overnight processing allows for optimal preparation of the biopsies and improved histological analysis. Artifacts that may be commonly encountered and can lead to interpretive difficulties include compression from the biotome, acute hemorrhage related to the procedure, and artifactual contraction-band change that is present in all biopsies.

M.C. Fishbein, MD
Department of Pathology and Laboratory Medicine,
David Geffen School of Medicine at the University of California,
Los Angeles, Los Angeles, CA, USA
e-mail: mfishbein@mednet.ucla.edu

© Springer International Publishing Switzerland 2016
W.D. Wallace, B.V. Naini (eds.), *Practical Atlas of Transplant Pathology*, DOI 10.1007/978-3-319-23054-2_2

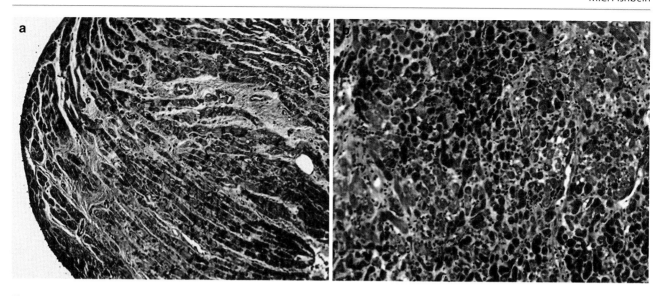

Fig. 2.1 Contraction-band artifact. Longitudinal (**a**) and cross-sectional (**b**) views of myocytes with contraction-band artifact. The contraction bands cause more and less eosinophilic regions that can mimic myocytolysis and/or coagulation necrosis

2.2 Acute Rejection

2.2.1 Acute Cell-Mediated Rejection (Figs. 2.2, 2.3, 2.4, and 2.5)

When cardiac transplantation was in its infancy, approximately 50 % of patients developed a hemodynamically significant episode of rejection during the first year after transplantation. Currently, at our institution, hemodynamically significant ACR occurs in less than 5 % of patients.

As with other solid organs, ACR in the transplanted heart is mediated by host cytotoxic and helper T-cells targeting graft antigens. One would therefore expect that T-lymphocytes would be the most numerous cells observed in the biopsy during an episode of rejection. In fact, our studies have shown that actually macrophages predominate. Usually, more than 50 % of the infiltrating cells are macrophages [2]. This finding turns out to be useful if IHC studies are performed to assist in the diagnosis of rejection versus QL. In ACR, most infiltrating cells will be macrophages with fewer T-lymphocytes and rare B-lymphocytes. In QL, most infiltrating cells will be B- or T-lymphocytes (depending on whether the top [B-cells] or bottom [T-cells] of the QL is biopsied, with only a relatively small proportion of macrophages. My personal practice is to order CD3, CD20, and CD68 on all biopsies suspected to have more than just mild rejection (grade 2R or 3R). C4d and CD31 (or 34) are also part of the package, as these immunostains are important in the evaluation of AMR to be discussed in a separate section.

In ACR, the first change noted is a perivascular infiltrate of mononuclear cells. These cells then spread out away from small blood vessels to involve interstitial tissue. As the ACR becomes more severe, myocyte injury becomes evident. Myocyte injury takes the form of coagulation necrosis only in very severe rejection. The more typical finding is that of "myocytolysis." Affected myocytes will lose their sarcoplasmic organelles and the sarcoplasm appears empty. Nuclei enlarge and nucleoli become prominent. Atrophy of myocytes is also observed. These injured myocytes are not necessarily irreversibly injured and they may recover. Interestingly, after injury, the affected fibers demonstrate a fetal phenotype. By IHC, they express vimentin and smooth muscle actin, proteins that are not expressed in normal adult cardiac myocytes.

Probably all transplanted hearts at some time demonstrate some rejection of some degree. The pathologist must not only identify ACR but also grade the findings. The pioneering work in this regard was done by Dr. Margaret Billingham and colleagues [3] at Stanford, who devised the first grading system. There have been several grading systems since, but remarkably, the current system in use to diagnose ACR is very similar to Dr. Billingham's first system.

Table 2.1 shows the criteria of grading for the current and most recent previous grading systems [4, 5]. The template we use at UCLA for reporting biopsy findings shows the criteria for each grade in both systems (See Appendix). We report both primarily for research purposes. The grade of rejection is based on the pattern of infiltrating cells and whether or not myocyte injury is present. This sounds easy, but artifacts in the tissue and lesions other than rejection can confound the interpretation.

- Grade 0R (no ACR) is diagnosed when there is no inflammatory infiltrate and no myocyte injury. Rare interstitial or perivascular lymphocytes may be present.
- Grade 1R (mild ACR) demonstrates focal perivascular infiltrates alone (previous 1A) or with some interstitial infiltrate as well (previous 1B) with no myocyte injury. A single focus of prominent cell infiltration that may be associated with myocyte injury is also considered grade 1R. This particular lesion was grade 2 in prior grading schemes. However, our studies, and those of others, have shown that these lesions are not rejection, but QLs [6]. This topic is still debated and some centers still regard these lesions as representing rejection.
- Grade 2R (moderate ACR), former grade 3A, is defined by two or more foci of cellular infiltrates with myocyte injury. The important distinguishing feature of grade 2R ACR is multifocal myocyte injury that is not present in grade 1R (prior 1B) ACR.
- Grade 3R (severe ACR) incorporates prior grades 3B and 4, and is characterized by diffuse inflammatory cell infiltrates that often contain eosinophils and neutrophils as well as lymphocytes and macrophages. Interstitial edema, hemorrhage, and vasculitis may be present, but in our experience, these findings are rare and more often observed in severe AMR. The difference between 2R and 3R is only the intensity and diffuseness of the process. The distinction is not critical, as in most transplant centers, both lesions are treated with augmentation of immunosuppression whether or not the patient is symptomatic or demonstrating graft dysfunction.

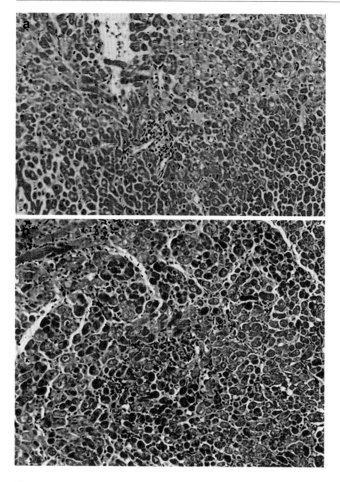

Fig. 2.2 Grade 1R ACR. (**a**) Prior grade 1A consists of a perivascular infiltrate of mononuclear cells. (**b**) Prior grade 1B shows mild interstitial as well as perivascular infiltration

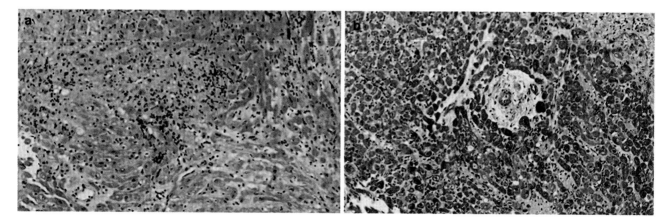

Fig. 2.3 Grade 2R ACR (prior grade 3A). (**a**, **b**) Multifocal mononuclear cell infiltrates with myocyte injury

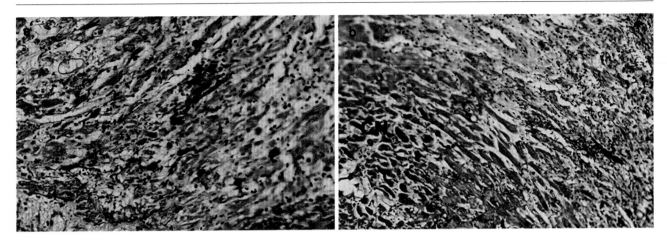

Fig. 2.4 Grade 3R ACR. (**a**, **b**) Prior grade 3B with diffuse interstitial infiltrates with myocyte injury. (**b**) Prior grade 4. Note diffuse infiltrates, interstitial hemorrhage, and extensive myocyte injury. Areas with coagulation necrosis (*CN*)

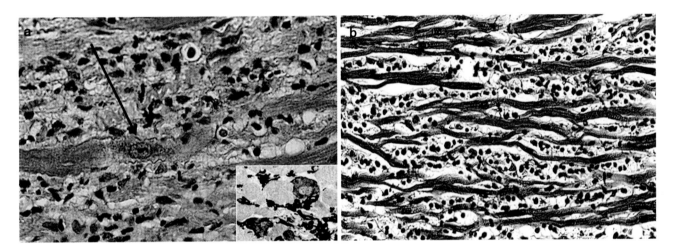

Fig. 2.5 Myocyte injury: examples of myocyte changes associated with injury. (**a**) Clearing of sarcoplasm and enlarged nucleus with prominent nucleolus (*arrow*). (**b**) Marked atrophy. *Inset*, Vimentin immunoperoxidase stain

Table 2.1 Acute cell-mediated rejection [5]

Grade 0 R	No evidence of cell-mediated rejection
Grade 1 R, mild	Interstitial and/or perivascular infiltrate with up to 1 focus of myocyte injury
	Previous grade 1A: Perivascular infiltrates without myocyte injury
	Previous grade 1B: Perivascular and sparse interstitial infiltrates without myocyte injury
Grade 2 R, moderate	Two or more foci of infiltrate with associated myocyte damage
	Previous grade 3A: Multifocal prominent infiltrates and/or myocyte injury
Grade 3 R, severe	Diffuse infiltrate with multifocal myocyte damage ± edema ± hemorrhage ± vasculitis
	Previous grade 3B: Diffuse infiltrates with myocyte injury
	Previous grade 4: Diffuse polymorphous infiltrate with myocyte injury ± hemorrhage ± edema ± vasculitis

2.2.2 Antibody-Mediated Rejection (Figs. 2.6, 2.7, 2.8, and 2.9)

AMR in cardiac transplantation was unrecognized for many years, and underrecognized for many more. Dr. Elizabeth Hammond and colleagues [7] at the University of Utah deserves credit for describing the clinical and pathological findings of AMR and emphasizing the importance of AMR. Before this work, the very existence of AMR had been questioned by prominent cardiac transplant physicians, including pathologists.

In AMR, graft injury results from antibodies, usually directed against antigens on endothelial cells that may initiate complement activation. With the decreasing incidence of ACR, AMR is now more common, affecting 10–20 % of patients, depending on the transplantation population. AMR is more common in "sensitized" patients, such as multiparous females, patients with prior blood transfusions, and those who have had implanted ventricular-assist devices. Typically, AMR is seen soon after transplantation in sensitized individuals, but can occur months or years later, especially in patients with no prior sensitization. AMR can cause

hemodynamic dysfunction, accelerated allograft vasculopathy, graft loss, and death.

The histological hallmark of AMR is dilation of capillaries by intraluminal cells that has been described as "endothelial swelling." Electron microscopic and IHC studies have shown that the majority of these cells are actually macrophages and not endothelial cells [8]. In addition to clarifying the nature of the process, this recognition is of practical importance; demonstrating intravascular macrophages by IHC staining is very helpful in making the diagnosis of AMR. CD31 or CD34 staining highlights capillary dilation and confirms the intravascular location of these cells, as opposed to the predominantly perivascular location of infiltrating cells in ACR.

C4d and/or C3d staining on capillaries that demonstrates complement deposition, can further confirm the diagnosis. Because the histological findings of AMR can be very subtle, sometimes the only evidence of AMR is by IF or IHC studies; therefore, it is recommended that these studies be done routinely early after transplantation or if the patient has unexplained cardiac dysfunction (Tables 2.2 and 2.3) [9].

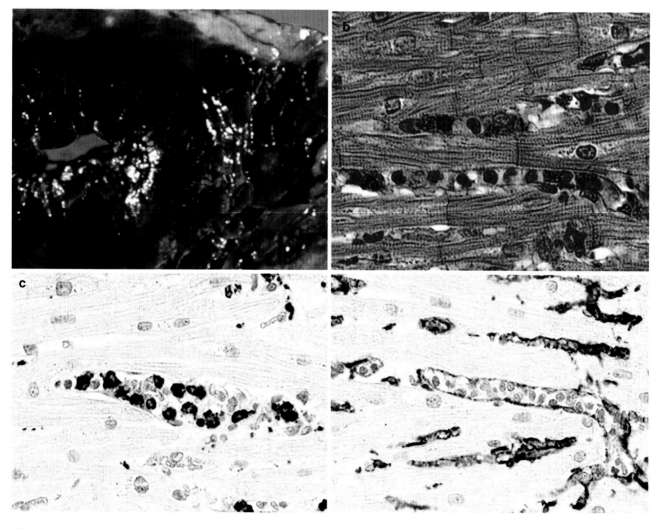

Fig. 2.6 AMR. (**a**) Gross photograph of a patient who died in cardiogenic shock 7 days after transplantation. Note hemorrhagic necrosis of the myocardium. (**b**) Note intravascular mononuclear cells. (**c**) CD68 immunostain confirms the presence of intravascular macrophages. (**d**) CD31 stain confirms the intracapillary location of macrophages

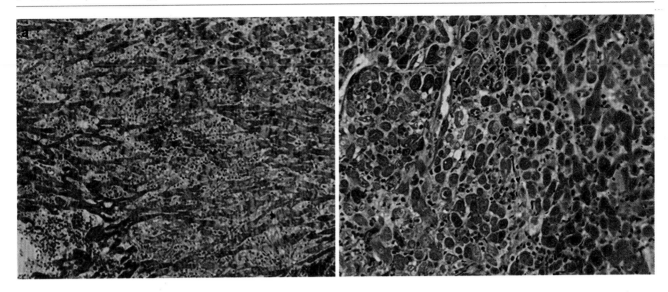

Fig. 2.7 AMR. (**a**, **b**) Low-power views show a hint of AMR because the interstitium is more cellular than normal, but they do not show clusters of lymphoid cells

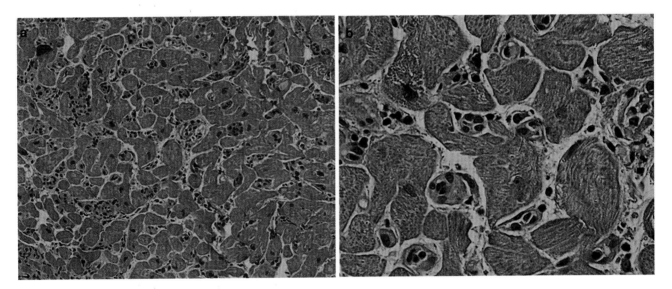

Fig. 2.8 AMR. (**a**) Low-power view shows interstitial mononuclear cells. (**b**) High magnification shows that the mononuclear cells are within, not around, the capillaries

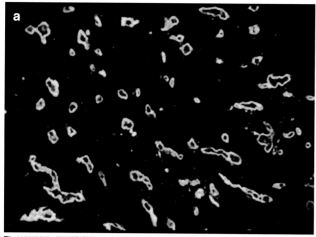

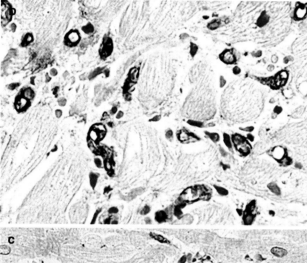

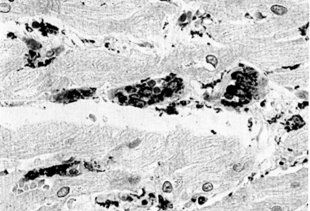

Fig. 2.9 AMR IH. Examples of IHC findings in AMR. (**a**) Positive IF staining for C4d in capillaries. (**b**) Positive immunoperoxidase staining for C4d in capillaries. (**c**) Positive IHC staining for macrophages (CD68) within capillaries

Table 2.2 Pathological diagnosis of AMR [9]

Macrophage accumulation in capillaries with distension of lumens
Endothelial cells may be prominent
In severe AMR, there is edema, hemorrhage, mixed inflammatory cell infiltrates, and myocyte necrosis
Intracapillary deposition of complement by IF or IHC
Intracapillary demonstration of macrophages by IF or IHC

Focal, mild changes are generally considered negative; each laboratory must establish its own baseline of findings

Table 2.3 Classification of AMR according to 2013 ISHLT working formulation [9]

pAMR0	Negative for AMR
	Histological and immunopathological findings are negative
pAMR 1 (H+)	Histological AMR alone
	Immunopathological findings are negative
pAMR 1 (I+)	Immunopathological alone
	CD68 + and/or C4d
pAMR 2 (H+, I+)	Histological and immunopathological studies both positive
pAMR 3	Severe AMR
	Histopathological and immunopathological findings plus edema, injury, and cell-mediated infiltrates

ISHLT International Society for Heart and Lung Transplantation

2.3 Other Pathological Entities in Endomyocardial Biopsy

2.3.1 Quilty Lesions (Figs. 2.10, 2.11, and 2.12)

QL is a peculiar endocardial infiltrate named by Dr. Billingham for the first patient in whom it was observed. QL has had other names as well. QL has been called "cyclosporine effect" because QL was not observed before the use of this immunosuppressive drug. QL is not considered to be "rejection" in that it is not associated with graft dysfunction, and if untreated, QL does not progress to histological or clinical manifestations of rejection. The pathogenesis is uncertain. The importance of QL is that it can be mistaken for rejection, resulting in unnecessary and potentially harmful treatment for rejection. The QL "A" is a flat or nodular infiltrate of mononuclear cells associated with microvascular proliferation, affecting the endocardium only. Eosinophils and plasma cells are often present. When QLs extend into the underlying myocardium, these are called QL "B." When this occurs, there may be associated myocyte injury. Recognizing the trabeculation of the subendocardial myocardium, and the potential for tangential sectioning of endomyocardial biopsies, it is quite possible that in a microscopic section of an endomyocardial biopsy, a QL B may appear to be purely intramyocardial. Accordingly, the appearance of an intramyocardial infiltrate with associated myocyte injury can lead to a misdiagnosis of ACR. Fortunately, IHC studies are quite useful in distinguishing QLs rich in B cells with few macrophages, from ACR, rich in macrophages with few B cells. One caveat is that in the deepest portion of QL Bs, the part in the myocardium, the immunophenotype of the lesion changes and is more like that of rejection with fewer B-lymphocytes and more macrophages.

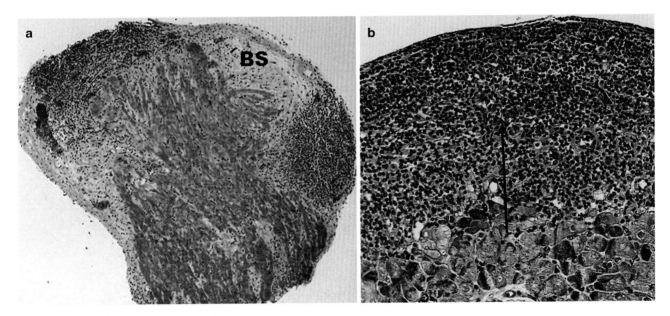

Fig. 2.10 QL B. (**a**) Note the prominent nodular endocardial infiltrate extending into the underlying myocardium, involving a healed biopsy site (BS). (**b**) A degenerating myocyte (*arrow*) may be seen in QL Bs

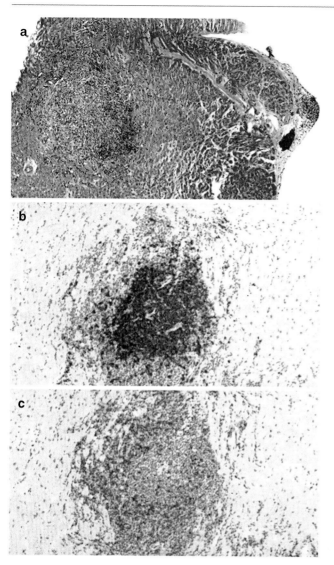

Fig. 2.11 QL B. QL B presenting as focal myocardial infiltrate. Immunostaining confirms that the lesion is not rejection. (**a**) Infiltrate appears intramyocardial. (**b**) CD20 stain demonstrates numerous B-lymphocytes. (**c**) CD68 stain demonstrates fewer macrophages

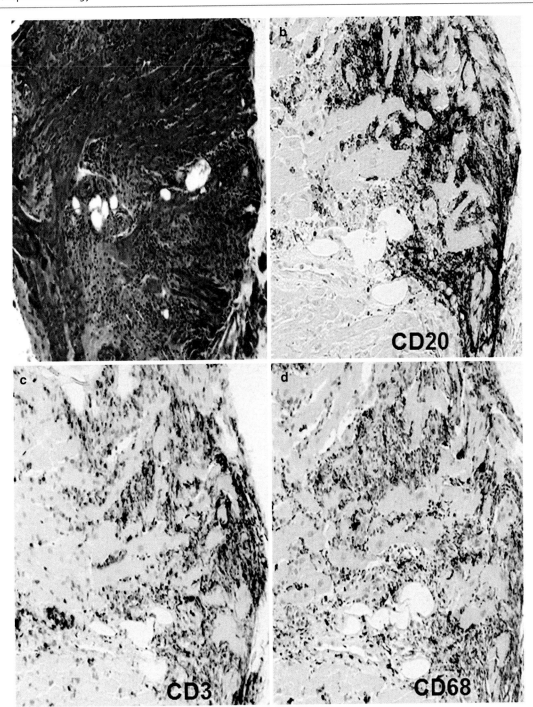

Fig. 2.12 Example of the usefulness of IHC staining in the evaluation for rejection. (**a**) Cellular-mediated infiltrate in a tangential section of endocardium and myocardium that could be ACR or a QL. Immunostaining establishes that this is a QL. (**b**) CD20 positive in a majority of infiltrating cells. (**c**) CD3 positive in fewer cells. (**d**) CD68 positive in a minority of cells

2.3.2   Ischemic Changes (Fig. 2.14)

If at the time of harvesting and implanting the donor heart, there is hypoxic injury to the myocardium, irreversible coagulation necrosis may occur. Because biopsies are typically not done until 1 or more weeks after transplantation, in addition to hypereosinophilia, loss of nuclei and other changes of coagulation necrosis of myocytes, including inflammatory/reparative changes, may be present. These include inflammation, granulation tissue proliferation, and/or collagen deposition. The changes of coagulation necrosis may be subtle. If the changes of coagulation necrosis are not appreciated, the inflammatory/reparative changes could be misinterpreted as a manifestation of rejection. If ischemic injury is observed, it should be noted in the pathology report, because this "nonimmune" injury is associated with more episodes of acute rejection, accelerated allograft vasculopathy, and early graft failure. Of note, owing to loss of membrane integrity, necrotic myocytes will take up plasma proteins nonspecifically. Accordingly, if IF studies are performed, these necrotic fibers will stain positively for a variety of plasma proteins, including immunoglobulins and complement components.

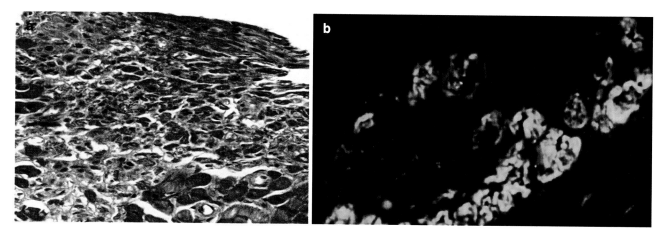

Fig. 2.13 Ischemic injury. (**a**) Region of subacute ischemic injury in a heart biopsy performed 1 week after transplantation. There is granulation tissue proliferation in addition to myocytes with coagulation necrosis. (**b**) IF study shows nonspecific C4d uptake in necrotic myocytes

2.3.3 Post-transplant Infections (Figs. 2.14, 2.15, and 2.16)

Unlike other transplanted solid organs, the lung, for example, infections in the transplanted heart are rare. The most common possibilities include cytomegalovirus, toxoplasmosis, and Chagas disease. Chagas disease may be present in the donor heart from donors who lived in endemic regions or it can involve the donor heart if the recipient was infected prior to transplantation. Both scenarios may occur.

The clue to Chagas disease of the heart is an eosinophilic myocarditis. Amastigotes within myocytes are visible in H&E-stained sections in fewer than half the cases and are difficult to find. There are IHC stains available, but they are virtually always negative if the organisms are not seen in H&E-stained sections. There are polymerase chain reactions (PCR) techniques that are more sensitive but not readily available. Tissue sections and blocks may be sent to the U.S. Centers for Disease Control and Prevention (CDC) for evaluation.

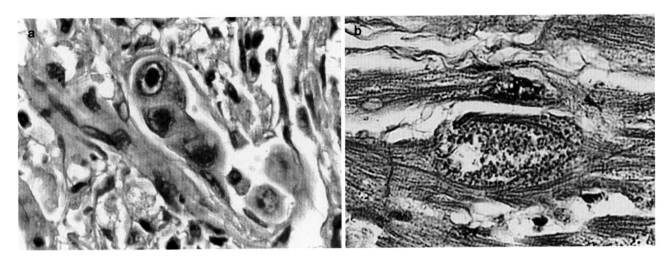

Fig. 2.14 Infections. (**a**) Cytomegalovirus with intranuclear inclusions in endothelial cells. (**b**) Chagas disease with amastigotes within myocytes

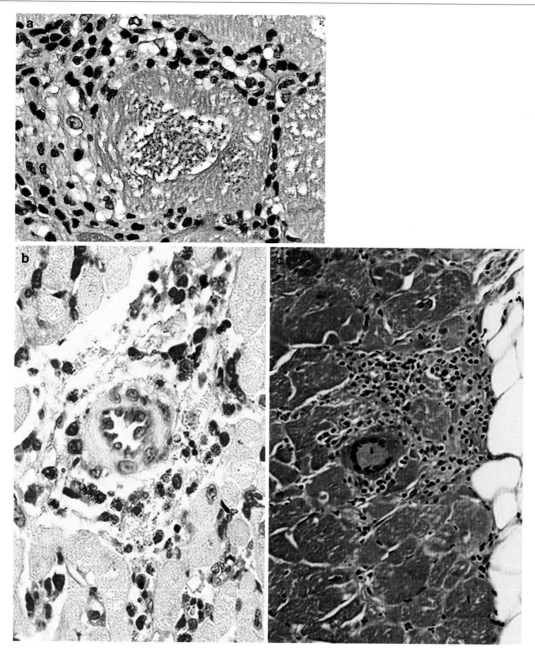

Fig. 2.15 Chagas disease. (**a**), Intracellular amastigotes surrounded by lymphocytic infiltrate. (**b**) Eosinophilic myocarditis (Giemsa stain). (**c**) Multinucleated giant cell that can be present

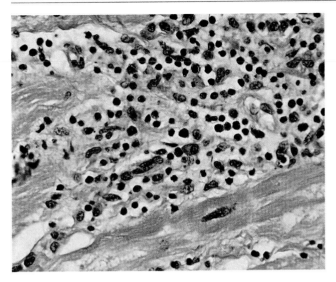

Fig. 2.16 Eosinophils. Eosinophils may be present in cell-mediated rejection, infections, and hypersensitivity myocarditis

2.3.4 Post-transplant Lymphoproliferative Disorders (Fig. 2.17)

PTLD is rare in the transplanted heart, but does occur. PTLD is manifest as an intense mononuclear cell infiltrate that resembles a QL B. The clue to the diagnosis of PTLD is that the lesion is much more infiltrative than a QL. The infiltrating lymphocytes may be atypical but, more often, are quite plasmacytoid. Immunostaining for CD20, CD138, and EBV usually resolves the issue. See Chap. 9 for more information.

Fig. 2.17 PTLD. (**a**), Endocardial
lymphocytes infiltrating the
underlying myocardium. (**b**)
Plasmacytoid appearance of some
of the lymphoid cells. (**c**) IHC stain
for kappa light chain is positive.
(**d**) Staining for lambda light chain
is negative

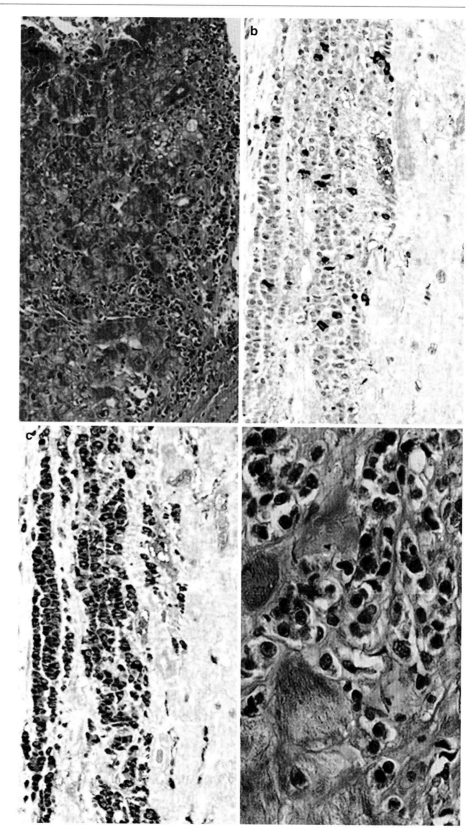

2.3.5 Prior Biopsy Sites (Fig. 2.18)

A very common finding in a patient who has had multiple biopsies is a previous biopsy site. The pathological findings will depend upon the time between biopsies. Early on, endocardial fibrin-rich deposits with organizational changes will dominate. Weeks later, only a scar will be observed. During healing, chronic inflammation may be prominent and suggestive of rejection. Biopsy sites typically contain prominent hemosiderin deposition and are well-demarcated "punched-out" lesions that involve the endocardium and myocardium. Therefore, rejection should not be diagnosed when inflammation is limited to connective tissue, as in a prior biopsy site, region of ischemic injury, or QL.

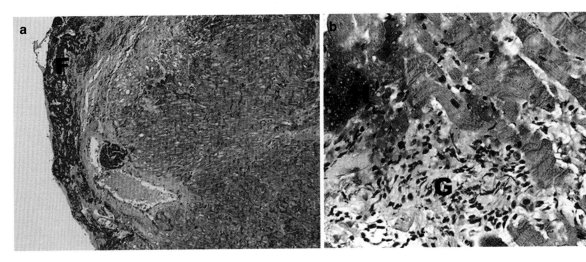

Fig. 2.18 Biopsy sites. (**a**), Recent biopsy site with fibrin deposition (*F*) on the endocardial surface. (**b**), Healing biopsy site consists of granulation tissue (*G*) with "crush artifact," a common artifact due to compression of the tissue by the bioptome. Acute hemorrhage related to the current procedure is also present (*H*)

2.3.6 Recurrent Disease in the Cardiac Allograft (Figs. 2.19 and 2.20)

Of course, the major concern in the evaluation of cardiac allografts is rejection. Confounding findings include technical artifacts, biopsy sites, QLs, PTLD, and infection. Another category of lesions that may be observed is recurrent cardiac disease in the allograft. Amyloidosis, Fabry disease, and sarcoidosis all may recur in the transplanted heart, but these should have no confusion with rejection. However, giant cell myocarditis, or eosinophilic myocarditis due to Chagas disease, or hypersensitivity myocarditis could easily be confused with rejection.

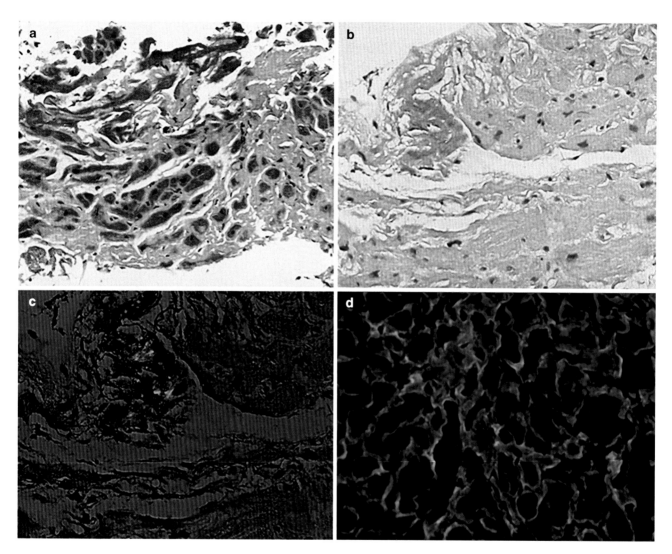

Fig. 2.19 Cardiac amyloidosis. Biopsy shows amorphous interstitial material (**a**) that stains positively with Congo red (**b**), has apple-green birefringence (**c**), and in this case, is positive for lambda light chains (**d**)

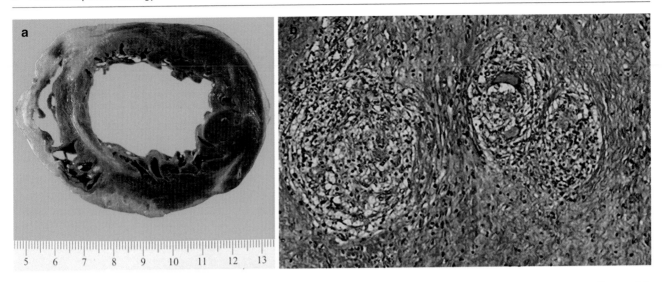

Fig. 2.20 Cardiac sarcoidosis. (**a**), Typical gross finding of scars in unusual locations in a young patient with no coronary artery disease; (**b**), Characteristic discrete non-necrotizing granulomata

2.4   Findings in the Explanted Transplanted Heart

It is not surprising that, when the pathologist has the entire heart, as opposed to small biopsies, more rejection is likely to be encountered. The grading system, accordingly, should not be used when reporting findings in the explanted heart. Descriptive terms such as mild, moderate, and severe are appropriate. In addition to changes noted in the myocardium, there will often be profound vascular changes in blood vessels not sampled during routine endomyocardial biopsy.

2.4.1   Cardiac Allograft Vasculopathy (Figs. 2.21, 2.22, 2.23, 2.24, and 2.25)

Virtually all transplanted hearts will demonstrate lymphocytes and macrophages in the intima of large arteries just beneath the endothelial layer ("endothelitis"), whether or not there is luminal narrowing. Cardiac allograft vasculopathy

(CAV) may be considered a form of arteriosclerosis that is a manifestation of chronic allograft rejection [10]. The process affects epicardial and intramyocardial arteries and veins as well. Typical atherosclerotic plaques with or without thrombosis may be seen in large and small epicardial arteries, but an obstructive fibromuscular intimal proliferation with or without evidence of arteritis in epicardial and myocardial arteries is a more characteristic finding. An important feature of CAV is the concentric and diffuse nature of the lesion in the vessels; this feature makes CAV more difficult to diagnose by standard coronary angiography. Hence, patients clinically thought to be free of CAV may suffer unexpected myocardial infarction or sudden cardiac death soon after a "negative" coronary angiogram. Intravascular ultrasound is considered to be a much more accurate technique for evaluation of CAV. A number of immune and nonimmune factors have been shown to play a role in the progression of CAV, which is the major factor limiting the long-term success of cardiac transplantation (Table 2.4). Statin drugs have been shown to slow, but not prevent, CAV.

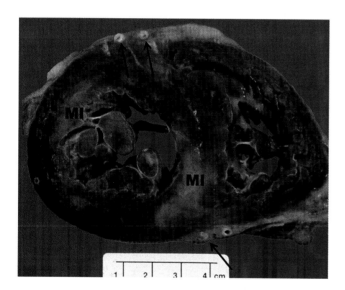

Fig. 2.21 CAV. Gross photograph shows arteries with abnormally thickened walls (*arrows*) and old, healed myocardial infarction (*MI*)

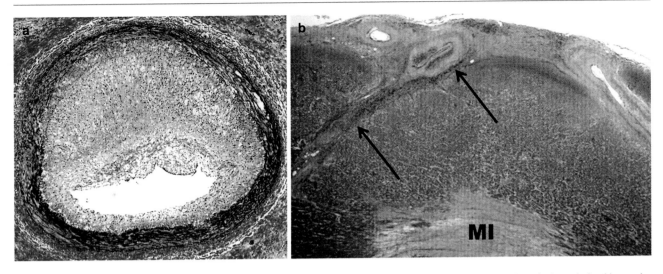

Fig. 2.22   CAV. (**a**), Eccentric atheroma in epicardial artery. (**b**), Section of epicardial artery with intramyocardial branch shows intimal hyperplasia and inflammation indicative of arteritis (*arrows*); an old healed *MI* is present

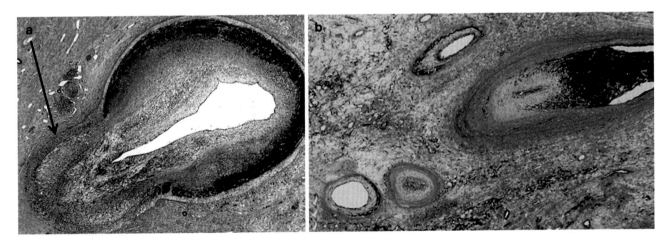

Fig. 2.23   CAV. (**a**) Epicardial coronary artery with intimal proliferation and evidence of past arteritis of media in a branch artery that caused loss of medial smooth muscle cells (*arrow*). (**b**) Epicardial arteries with intimal proliferation and organizing thrombus (*T*)

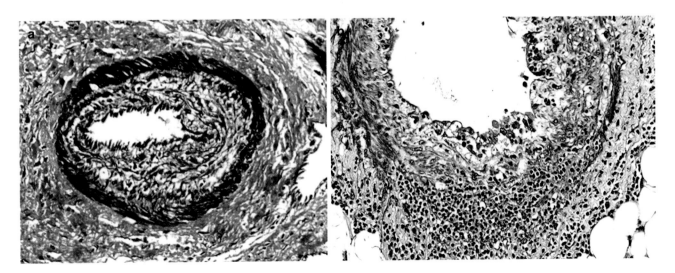

Fig. 2.24   CAV involving intramyocardial arteries. Fibromuscular intimal hyperplasia (**a**) with arteritis (**b**) as well

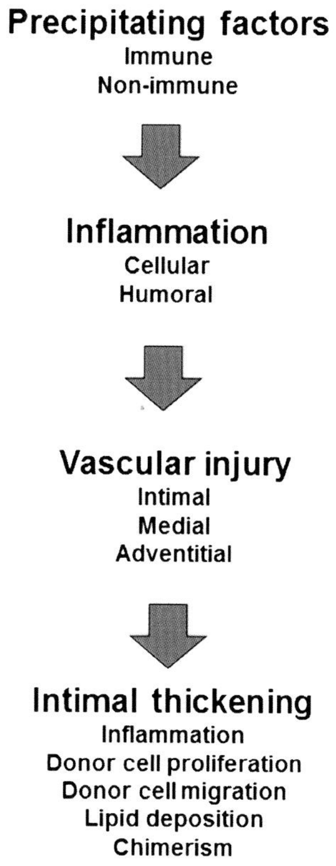

Precipitating factors
Immune
Non-immune

Inflammation
Cellular
Humoral

Vascular injury
Intimal
Medial
Adventitial

Intimal thickening
Inflammation
Donor cell proliferation
Donor cell migration
Lipid deposition
Chimerism

Fig. 2.25 Diagram of proposed pathogenesis of CAV

Table 2.4 Risk factors for CAV

Cell-mediated rejection	Number and severity of episodes
AMR	Number and severity of episodes
Ischemia/reperfusion injury	Duration of ischemia prior to transplantation
Infections	Most notably cytomegalovirus
Medications	Such as steroids
Risk factors for atherosclerosis	Smoking, hyperlipidemia, diabetes, etc.

References

1. Chantranuwat C, Qiao JH, Kobashigawa J, Hong L, Shintaku P, Fishbein MC. Immunoperoxidase staining for C4d on paraffin-embedded tissue in cardiac allograft endomyocardial biopsies: comparison to frozen tissue immunofluorescence. Appl Immunohistochem Mol Morphol. 2004;12:166–71.

2. Michaels PJ, Espejo ML, Kobashigawa J, Alejos JC, Burch C, Takemoto S, et al. Humoral rejection in cardiac transplantation: risk factors, hemodynamic consequences and relationship to transplant coronary artery disease. J Heart Lung Transplant. 2003;22:58–69.

3. Billingham ME, Cary NR, Hammond ME, Kemnitz J, Marboe C, McCallister HA, et al. A working formulation for the standardization of nomenclature in the diagnosis of heart and lung rejection: Heart Rejection Study Group. The International Society for Heart Transplantation. J Heart Transplant. 1994;13:1051–7.

4. Berry GJ, Angelini A, Burke MM, Bruneval P, Fishbein MC, Hammond E, et al. The ISHLT working formulation for pathologic diagnosis of antibody-mediated rejection in heart transplantation: evolution and current status (2005–2011). J Heart Transplant. 2011;6:601–11.

5. Stewart S, Winters GL, Fishbein MC, Tazelaar HD, Kobashigawa J, Abrams J, et al. Revision of the 1990 working formulation for the standardization of nomenclature in the diagnosis of heart rejection. J Heart Lung Transplant. 2005;24:1710–20.

6. Fishbein MC, Bell G, Lones MA, Czer LS, Miller JM, Harasty D, et al. Grade 2 cell-mediated heart rejection: does it exist? J Heart Lung Transplant. 1994;13:1051–7.

7. Hammond EH, Yowell RL, Nunoda S, Menlove RL, Renlund DG, Bristow MR, et al. Vascular (humoral) rejection in heart transplantation: pathologic observations and clinical implications. J Heart Transplant. 1989;8:430–43.

8. Lones MA, Czer LS, Trento A, Harasty D, Miller JM, Fishbein MC. Clinical-pathologic features of humoral rejection in cardiac allografts: a study in 81 consecutive patients. J Heart Lung Transplant. 1995;14:151–62.

9. Berry GJ, Burke MM, Anderson C, Bruneval P, Fedrigo M, Fishbein MC, et al. The 2013 International Society for Heart and Lung Transplantation Working Formulation for the standardization of nomenclature in the pathologic diagnosis of antibody-mediated rejection in heart transplantation. J Heart Lung Transplant. 2013;32:1147–62.

10. Lu W-H, Palatnik K, Fishbein GA, Lai C, Levi DS, Perens G, et al. Diverse morphologic manifestations of cardiac allograft vasculopathy: a pathologic study of 64 allograft hearts. J Heart Lung Transplant. 2011;30:1044–50.

Lung Transplant Pathology

3

W. Dean Wallace and Carol F. Farver

Pathological evaluation of lung allograft specimens presents several challenges unique to lung transplant patients. Through the airways, the lungs communicate directly with the outside world and pathology specimens may include aerosolized exogenous particulate matter or organisms that are not otherwise encountered in other solid organ transplants. Furthermore, owing to interruption of the lower vagal nerve fibers during the transplantation procedure, the cough reflex is diminished in lung transplant patients resulting in increased risk for aspiration, leading to bacterial pneumonia or aspirated foreign material causing low-level chronic or acute inflammation that could cause interpretive difficulties for the pathologist [1].

The transbronchial biopsy remains the major tool used to monitor for allograft rejection of the transplanted lung. It usually consists of only a few small portions of alveolar tissue that are easily crushed and distorted by the biopsy procedure. This artifactual distortion can render interpretation extremely difficult or impossible. In these areas of crush artifact, some findings, such as inflammation, often cannot be localized and essentially must be ignored. The exception to this rule is the discovery of organisms or neoplastic cells, which should always be reported. However, even the discovery of some organisms, such as *Aspergillus*, may be inconclusive as to the characteristic of the infection (e.g., is the organism invasive or colonizing an airway?) In this situation, correlation with clinical findings and discussion with the bronchoscopist may be most helpful.

For complete diagnostic evaluation, correlation with concurrent clinical information is necessary. This is necessary because features of infection and acute rejection have considerable histological overlap. The overall diagnostic interpretation may be quite different in a 30-year-old man who had recently lost his insurance and has not been taking anti-rejection medication versus a 50-year-old man who has been taking his medication but has had recent contact with sick people infected with adenovirus or cytomegalovirus (CMV), yet the pathological features on a small transbronchial biopsy may be quite similar in areas. The presence of convincing perivascular lymphoid infiltrates with endotheliitis should strongly indicate the diagnosis of rejection; identification of the pathogen, in this case a viral inclusion, would confirm the infection. The finding of both features of rejection and organisms would indicate infection; concurrent rejection would require clinical correlation and judgment.

3.1 Pathological Rejection Classification

The most commonly used system for evaluating lung transplant transbronchial biopsies is the most recent International Society of Heart and Lung Transplant (ISHLT) classification [2]. The ISHLT classification of acute rejection in the lung transplant is based on the presence, intensity, and distribution of mononuclear cell infiltration in the alveolar parenchyma and any accompanying acute lung injury. The grading system ranges from A0 (none) to A4 (severe). Airway inflammation is graded from B0 (none) to B2R (high grade) and is based on intensity of mononuclear cell infiltration in the airway wall and presence or absence of mucosal injury. Chronic airway rejection is described as C0 (absent) or C1 (present) and is based on the presence of abnormal subepithelial fibrosis. Chronic vascular rejection, category D, is poorly defined in the lung, may be quite rare in the allograft, and, importantly, is difficult to interpret in small transbronchial biopsies. Therefore, it does not have a grading scheme in the ISHLT classification. In our practice, we tend to only diagnose chronic vascular rejection in allograft explant specimens or at autopsy where large areas of tissue allow for an optimal examination of the pulmonary vessels (Table 3.1).

W.D. Wallace, MD (✉)
Department of Pathology and Laboratory Medicine,
David Geffen School of Medicine at the University of California,
Los Angeles, 10833 Le Conte Avenue, 27-061C4 CHS,
Los Angeles, CA 90095-1732, USA
e-mail: wwallace@mednet.ucla.edu

C.F. Farver, MD
Pathology and Laboratory Medicine Institute, Cleveland Clinic,
Cleveland, OH, USA

© Springer International Publishing Switzerland 2016
W.D. Wallace, B.V. Naini (eds.), *Practical Atlas of Transplant Pathology*, DOI 10.1007/978-3-319-23054-2_3

Table 3.1 ISHLT lung allograft grading system, 2007 working formulation [2]

Acute rejection grade	
A0	No rejection
A1	Minimal rejection
A2	Mild rejection
A3	Moderate rejection
A4	Severe rejection
Airway inflammation grade	
B0	No significant inflammation
B1R	Low-grade inflammation
B2R	High-grade inflammation
BX	Ungradeable
Chronic airway rejection grade	
C0	Not present
C1	Present

3.1.1 Acute Rejection

3.1.1.1 Grade A0

No rejection; there are no significant perivascular inflammatory cell infiltrates. The presence of a few small noncircumferential infiltrates is not sufficient for a diagnosis of A1 (Figs. 3.1 and 3.2).

3.1.1.2 Grade A1

Minimal rejection; there are scattered and infrequent perivascular mononuclear cell infiltrates in alveolar tissue with only few eosinophils and no endotheliitis. The presence of endotheliitis would indicate at least grade A2 rejection. Some (if not all) infiltrates should be entirely circumferential around vessels. If many vessels are involved, this may not be "minimal" rejection and we tend to regard this as grade A2 (Figs. 3.3 and 3.4).

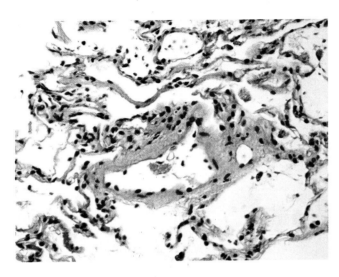

Fig. 3.1 Postcapillary venule with few scattered mononuclear cells, primarily lymphocytes, in adjacent interstitium. The sparse inflammatory cell infiltrate is not diagnostic of acute rejection

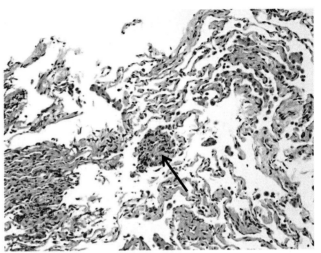

Fig. 3.3 Small lymphoid infiltrate centered on a postcapillary venule (*arrow*). Note the lumen containing red cells in the center of the picture. The alveolar tissue is mildly collapsed but the small perivascular infiltrate is distinct and entirely circumferential, indicating grade A1. There are no identifiable endotheliitis, eosinophils, or interstitial inflammation in alveolar walls

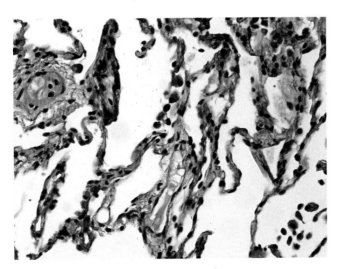

Fig. 3.2 Small postcapillary venule with few scattered neutrophils in nearby capillaries. This biopsy is 3 weeks post-transplant, and the mild neutrophilic infiltrate is normal in this setting

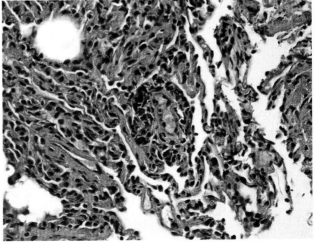

Fig. 3.4 Distinct lymphoid infiltrate centered on a postcapillary venule, consistent with grade A1. Despite the slight crush artifact, it is easy to see there are no identifiable endotheliitis, eosinophils, or interstitial inflammation in alveolar walls

3.1.1.3 Grade A2

Mild rejection; this grade is characterized by more frequent and larger perivascular chronic inflammatory cell infiltrates around venules and arterioles, often with accompanying eosinophils and endotheliitis. Venules appear to be more frequently involved than arterioles. The presence of only rare eosinophils is not sufficient to warrant a diagnosis of A2 rejection by itself, but it should prompt careful review of the biopsy material for more features of grade A2. Furthermore, the absence of endotheliitis does not exclude grade A2 rejection if other features are present. There is obviously room for interpretive differences in frequency and size of perivascular inflammatory cell infiltrates between grades A1 and A2; the ISHLT guidelines suggest the perivascular infiltrates of A2 are more easily recognizable at lower scanning power. This is fair advice, but experienced pathologists are able to detect small A1 perivascular infiltrates at low power and must be able to adjust their grading criteria accordingly (Figs. 3.5 and 3.6).

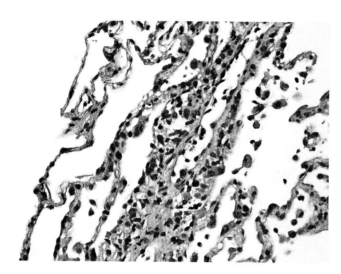 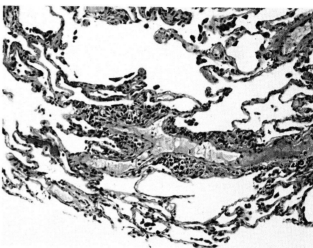

Fig. 3.5 Prominent mononuclear cell infiltrate around a venule and accompanying endothelial inflammation, consistent with grade A2. There are scattered inflammatory cells in nearby alveolar septa but there is no obvious expansion of the interstitial space

Fig. 3.6 Prominent mononuclear cell infiltrate around a venule and scattered eosinophils, consistent with grade A2. Similar to Fig. 3.5, there are scattered inflammatory cells in nearby alveolar septa but there is no obvious expansion of the interstitial space

3.1.1.4 Grade A3

Moderate rejection; this grade is defined by the extension of the inflammatory cell infiltrate into the alveolar septa. There are usually concurrent endotheliitis and frequent eosinophils but not always. There may be features of mild acute lung injury with fibrin deposition but there are no hyaline membranes (Figs. 3.7, 3.8, and 3.9).

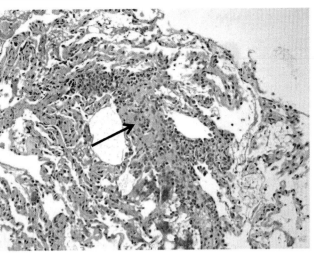

Fig. 3.9 Prominent mononuclear cell infiltrate around a venule with endotheliitis, few conspicuous eosinophils, and interstitial inflammation and expansion in adjacent alveolar septa, consistent with grade A3. The endotheliitis and intravascular inflammation is so prominent, it is difficult to discern the lumen of the vessel in the center of the picture (*arrow*)

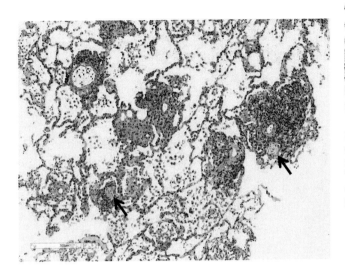

Fig. 3.7 Prominent mononuclear cell infiltrates around multiple vessels with interstitial inflammation and few small polyps of organizing pneumonia (*arrows*), consistent with grade A3

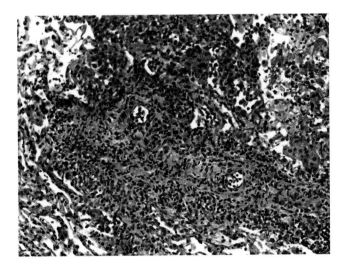

Fig. 3.8 Very prominent mononuclear cell infiltrate around a vessel with mixed interstitial inflammation, including eosinophils, and expansion from a case with grade A3

3.1.1.5 Grade A4

Severe rejection: this grade of rejection is characterized by concurrent severe acute lung injury with features of acute cellular rejection, specifically perivascular and interstitial mononuclear cell infiltrates with or without endotheliitis and eosinophils. The acute lung injury demonstrates hyaline membranes and reactive pneumocyte injury. Paradoxically, the rejection-associated inflammatory cell infiltrates may be diminished, compared with grade A3 or A2 rejection, and distinction from nonrejection causes of lung injury may be difficult. Pathological confirmation of perivascular infiltrates and exclusion of infection by special stains and/or microbiology studies, and clinical correlation are usually sufficient to confirm the diagnosis of severe rejection (Figs. 3.10, 3.11, and 3.12).

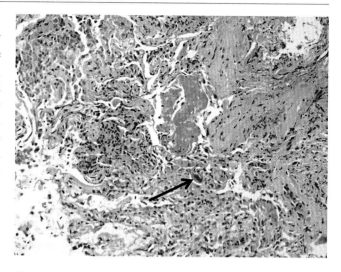

Fig. 3.11 Higher-power image of Fig. 3.10 reveals reactive pneumocyte changes within the severe acute lung injury. The large reactive nucleus with a purple hue (*arrow*) may raise concern for viral inclusion. However, this reactive pneumocyte with nucleomegaly is a mimicker for viral infection. Viral studies on this biopsy were negative; the patient had missed antirejection medications for several weeks and was clinically more likely to have rejection than infection. The etiology of the acute lung injury is still not apparent in this field of view

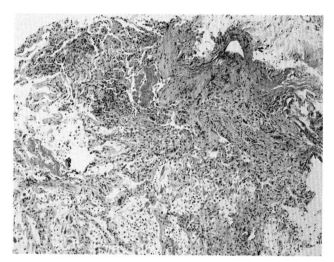

Fig. 3.10 Diffuse acute lung injury with fibrin deposition, interstitial and alveolar cellular infiltrates, and pneumocyte injury. Obvious biopsy distortion is appreciable at the top of the image; nevertheless, the severe and diffuse acute lung injury is readily apparent. The etiology of the acute lung injury is not obvious in this field of view

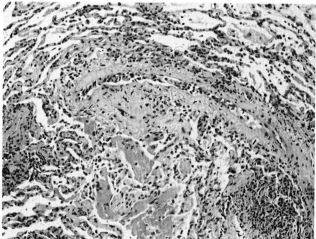

Fig. 3.12 On this area of the same biopsy from Figs. 3.10 and 3.11, a vessel with clear endotheliitis and mild perivascular and adjacent interstitial cellular infiltration is seen. These features are diagnostic of rejection. In the lower portion of the image, acute lung injury with fibrin deposition is seen; this corresponds to grade A4 rejection. Note the relative diminution of the cellular infiltrate in comparison with the images of A3 rejection. This case serves to demonstrate the importance of sufficient sampling, careful pathological review of the entire specimen, and clinical correlation before diagnosis is rendered

3.1.2 Airway Inflammation

The previous edition of the ISHLT lung transplant grading system divided airway inflammation into 5 grades, from B0 (no inflammation) to B4 (severe inflammation) [3]. To simplify the system and improve reproducibility among pathologists, the most recent ISHLT grading system collapsed the grades into 3 categories: B0 (no significant airway inflammation), B1R (low-grade bronchiolar inflammation), and B2R (high-grade bronchiolar inflammation). Grade B1R is a combination of previous grades B1 and B2; and grade B2R is a combination of previous grades B3 and B4. "R" is used to designate the revision and to avoid confusion with the previous grades. Grade BX is used to designate uninterpretable airways if the airways are not sampled, are distorted by crush or sectioning artifact, or if there is a concurrent infection causing airway inflammation.

3.1.2.1 Grade B0

No significant inflammation; there may be scattered chronic inflammatory cells associated with the small airways but the infiltrate would be within normal limits.

3.1.2.2 Grade B1R

Low-grade bronchiolar inflammation; there are varying degrees of mononuclear cells within the submucosa and muscular layers of the small airway. There may be mild lymphocytic infiltration of the epithelium but there is no significant epithelial cell injury. Small vessels around the airway may have circumferential perivascular infiltrates suggestive of acute rejection grade A1. If these vessels are part of the airway, the inflammation should be considered a component of the airway inflammation and not acute rejection (Figs. 3.13 and 3.14).

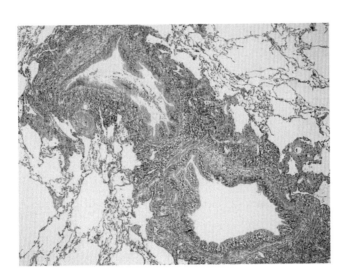

Fig. 3.13 Low-power view of a bronchiole with prominent circumferential mononuclear cell infiltrate including cellular infiltration within the deeper epithelium. There is no appreciable epithelial cell injury and this is most consistent with B1R

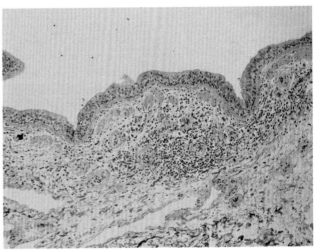

Fig. 3.14 The bronchiolar wall has a conspicuous mononuclear cell infiltrate in the deeper connective tissue. Note the involvement and inflammation of small vessels in the wall. There is mononuclear cell infiltration within the epithelium, but overall, the infiltrate is mild and the paucity of epithelial cell injury is most consistent with B1R

3.1.2.3 Grade B2R

High grade; this grade is characterized by more intense intraepithelial lymphocytic infiltration and epithelial cell injury manifesting as metaplasia or frank necrosis. Eosinophils are more common than in grade B1R. If there are abundant neutrophils, an infectious etiology should be considered and, if proven or favored, grade BX should be rendered (Figs. 3.15 and 3.16).

3.1.2.4 Grade BX

Ungradeable; when no airway is present on the biopsy or is obscured by handling artifact or infection-associated inflammation, this is designated as grade BX. Data from the Banff Study of Pathologic Findings Associated with HLA Antibodies found 38 % of cases, from a pool of 253 biopsies, were graded BX [4].

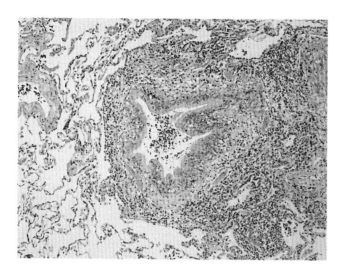

Fig. 3.15 This bronchiole shows very prominent circumferential mononuclear cell infiltration including cellular infiltration throughout the entire epithelium. There is disruption of the normal epithelial architecture with epithelial cell dehiscence in the areas of most prominent inflammation. Overall, the features are most consistent with B2R

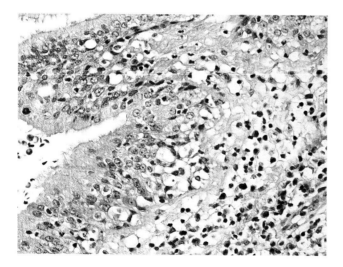

Fig. 3.16 High-power view of Fig. 3.15 in an area of epithelial inflammation and injury. Note the mixed cellular infiltrate including occasional neutrophils and eosinophils and the loss of normal epithelial architecture near the basement membrane. In this case, intact cilia may be seen in some areas; this does not preclude the presence of significant epithelial cell injury in deeper portions of the epithelium

3.2 Chronic Rejection/Chronic Lung Allograft Dysfunction

Chronic rejection of the lung allograft is the major cause of graft failure and death in lung transplant patients. Classically, chronic rejection has been recognized as the development of an obstructive defect termed bronchiolitis obliterans syndrome (BOS). As understanding and experience of chronic lung transplant rejection has increased, various phenotypes have been recognized and the term chronic lung allograft dysfunction (CLAD) has been coined to accommodate all forms of chronic allograft rejection in the lung [5]. All forms of CLAD are poorly demonstrated on transbronchial biopsies and are best evaluated with clinical and radiographic evaluation.

The pathological features are usually best seen on explant or autopsy specimens. Gross evaluation of explant specimens reveals fibrous adhesions to the chest wall or between lobes. On cross section, the pleura and interlobular septa are more prominent and fibrotic (Figs. 3.17 and 3.18).

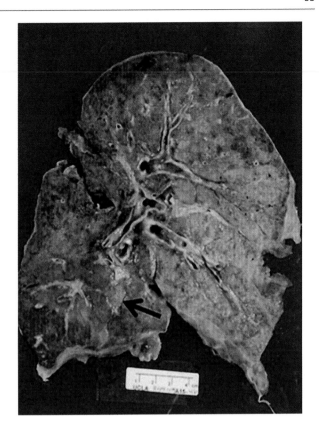

Fig. 3.18 Cross-section of the right lung allograft. Note the subtle accentuation of interlobular septa and pleural thickening, consistent with septal (*arrow*) and pleural fibrosis (Courtesy of Dr. Josephine Aguilar-Jakthong)

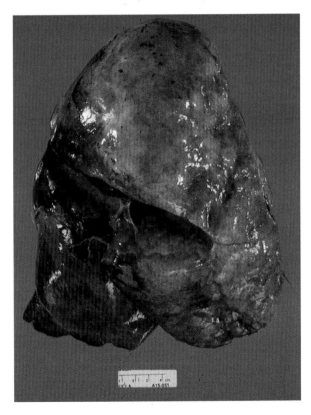

Fig. 3.17 External surface of a transplanted right lung at the time of autopsy. Note the adhesions between the middle and the upper lobes (Courtesy of Dr. Josephine Aguilar-Jakthong)

3.2.1 Bronchiolitis Obliterans

BOS manifests as a decrease in forced expiratory volume per 1 second (FEV_1), may result in eventual graft loss and contributes to the 5-year graft survival of approximately 50 % [6]. The development of BOS is not reliably evaluated by the transbronchial biopsy and is best monitored by clinical and radiological evaluation. Nevertheless, the presence of airway scarring, termed bronchiolitis obliterans (BO), should be reported if discovered on a transbronchial biopsy. If there is no evidence of airway scarring, the grade is C0; if scarring is present, the grade is C1. The scarring begins as subepithelial granulation tissue with small vessels within an edematous fibrous stroma. The process may be concentric or eccentric. Eventually, the granulation tissue is replaced by dense fibrous scar tissue that causes progressive obstruction of the small airways and may ultimately lead to complete obliteration. The findings may be difficult to appreciate on a hematoxylin and eosin (H&E) stain and the features can be highlighted with special connective tissue stains, such as Movat, Masson trichrome, or elastic stains (Figs. 3.19 and 3.20).

Distal to the lesion, postobstructive changes, such as clusters of foam cells or cholesterol clefts with granulomas, may be seen (Fig. 3.21). However, these are nonspecific findings and, although these features are suggestive, do not indicate a diagnosis of BO without sampling of the lesion in the airway. Pathological features of BO are more easily discovered in larger resection specimens such as allograft explants (Figs. 3.22 and 3.23).

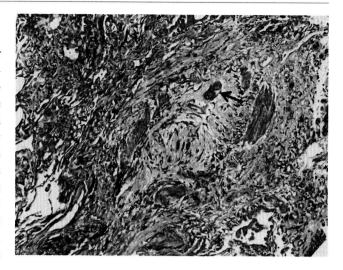

Fig. 3.20 Same area of bronchiolar wall from Fig. 3.19. Note the well-defined elastic layer within the smooth muscle bundles and the reactive fibrosis obliterating the airway. This is diagnostic of Bronchiolitis Obliterans (BO), or grade C1. Note the residual airway epithelium (*arrow*). This image demonstrates the value of special connective tissue stains (Combined Masson trichrome and elastic van Gieson stain)

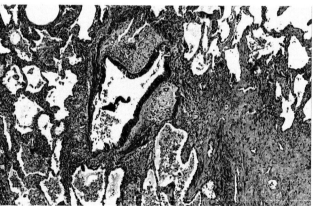

Fig. 3.21 Bronchiole with eccentric subepithelial fibrosis and postobstructive foamy macrophages in adjacent alveolar ducts and sacs; consistent with BO (Movat stain)

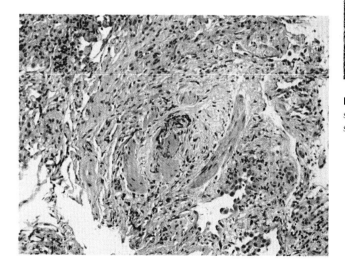

Fig. 3.19 Area of the bronchiolar wall with smooth muscle bundles, fibroconnective tissue, and mild nonspecific chronic inflammation. It is difficult to discern which part of the bronchiolar wall is pictured. There is no identifiable lumen and the smooth muscle bundles may be from an area of tangential sectioning. The rounding of the bundles of smooth muscle may be suggestive of an obliterated airway, but the diagnosis is difficult to confirm with this image

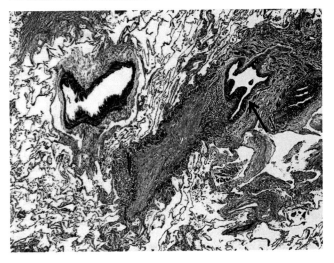

Fig. 3.22 Lung allograft explant specimen. Note the complete obliteration of the airway in the center of the image. A branch of the airway to the right of the area of obliteration appears to be uninvolved by BO (*arrow*) (Combined Masson trichrome and elastic van Gieson stain)

3.2.2 Chronic Vascular Rejection

As in other transplanted organs, larger vessels in the pulmonary allograft may be affected by chronic rejection. Both pulmonary arteries and pulmonary veins may be affected and the patients may develop pulmonary hypertension. At least one study has found a correlation between chronic vascular rejection and BOS, with ultimately increased risk for graft loss [7]. Like BO, the transbronchial biopsy is a very insensitive method for detecting chronic vascular rejection. However, the features of chronic vascular rejection are relatively specific and demonstrate intimal fibrosis with infiltration of mononuclear cells. The medial smooth muscle is often atrophied (Figs. 3.24, 3.25, 3.26, and 3.27).

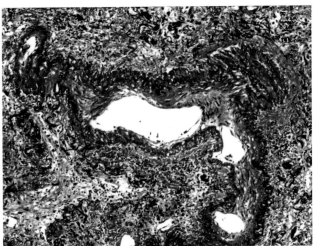

Fig. 3.24 Lung allograft explant specimen. This artery demonstrates irregular intimal fibrosis with scattered mononuclear cells throughout the intima. The smooth muscle in the media is indistinct and atrophied. Note the obliterated bronchiole in the bottom left of the picture (Combined Masson trichrome and elastic van Gieson stain)

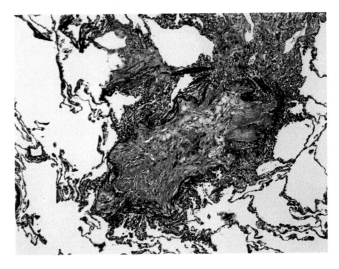

Fig. 3.23 Lung allograft explant specimen. This small airway is completely obliterated. The lumen is completely replaced by variably dense fibrosis with scattered mononuclear cells and few capillaries. The surrounding smooth muscle bundles are partially atrophied (Combined Masson trichrome and elastic van Gieson stain)

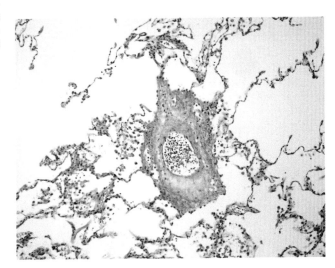

Fig. 3.25 Pulmonary vein with thickened fibrous wall, scattered mononuclear cells, and rare eosinophils. This is chronic rejection of a pulmonary vein vaguely resembling pulmonary veno-occlusive disease (PVOD)

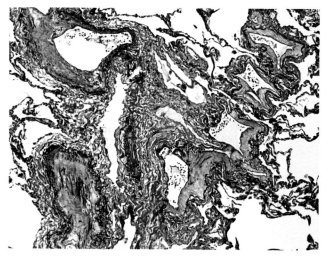

Fig. 3.26 Lung allograft explant specimen. This is chronic rejection of a pulmonary vein in a PVOD pattern. Note the waxy intimal fibrosis with scattered mononuclear cells (Combined Masson trichrome and elastic van Gieson stain)

3.2.3 Restrictive Allograft Syndrome

More recently, it has been recognized patients with CLAD with BOS may also demonstrate loss of total lung capacity (TLC) and radiographic features of interstitial lung disease with upper lobe predominance. This process is labeled restrictive allograft syndrome (RAS) and has been defined as CLAD with less than 90 % baseline TLC [8]. These patients appear to always have concurrent BOS. Pathologically, the interstitium and airspaces are filled with hyalinized fibrosis with scattered mononuclear cells. The fibrosis characteristically is most prominent at the periphery of the lungs and is difficult to sample with a transbronchial biopsy. Nevertheless, radiological correlation may help to explain irregular fibrosis sampled on a transbronchial biopsy (Figs. 3.28 and 3.29). Overall, the pathology is best demonstrated in larger biopsies or explant specimens (Figs. 3.30, 3.31, and 3.32).

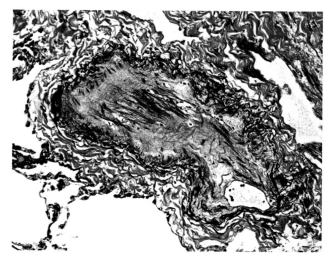

Fig. 3.27 Higher-power view of Fig. 3.26. Note the waxy intimal fibrosis with scattered mononuclear cells and smooth muscle atrophy in the media (Combined Masson trichrome and elastic van Gieson stain)

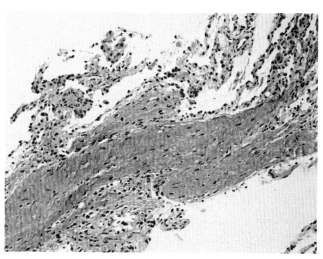

Fig. 3.28 Transbronchial biopsy with prominent area of dense hyalinized fibrosis. The area of fibrosis is much larger and more hyalinized than typical organizing pneumonia. Nevertheless, radiological and clinical correlations are necessary to confirm the diagnosis of RAS

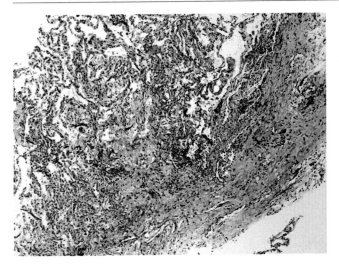

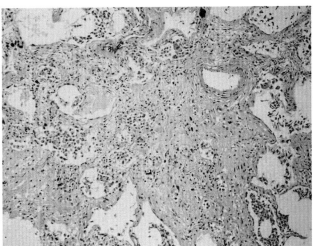

Fig. 3.29 Same biopsy as Fig. 3.28. This connective tissue stain better illustrates the interstitial fibrosis. In this picture, the fibrosis appears to be most prominent in a lobular septum (Combined Masson trichrome and elastic van Gieson stain)

Fig. 3.31 Same patient from Fig. 3.30. The patient from Fig. 3.30 unfortunately died and went to autopsy several weeks later. Unfortunately, several weeks later the patient from Fig. 3.30 died and went to autopsy. In this area, there is interstitial and airspace fibrosis with obvious architectural distortion

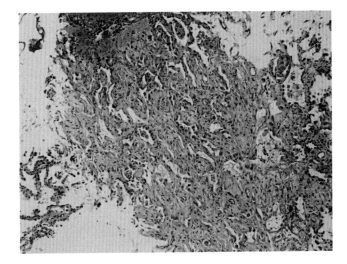

Fig. 3.30 Transbronchial biopsy with acute lung injury and interstitial widening with early fibrosis. At this time, the diagnosis of "acute and organizing lung injury" was given

Fig. 3.32 Peripheral lung from
case with RAS. (**a**) Note the
dense subpleural and septal
fibrosis. (**b**) At higher power,
note how the fibrosis appears to
fill in the alveolar spaces but
leaves the underlying alveolar
architecture intact. The elastic
tissue outlining the alveolar walls
is still present in most areas
(Movat stain)

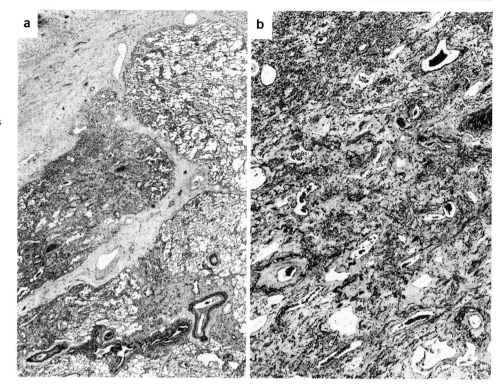

3.3   Neutrophilic Reversible Allograft Dysfunction

A newly described manifestation of CLAD is neutrophilic reversible allograft dysfunction (NRAD). This has been defined as 15 % or greater neutrophils in bronchiolar lavage (BAL) fluid in patients with diagnostic features of CLAD but no evidence of infection. Importantly, some studies have shown these patients have a good prognosis and respond to azithromycin with improvement of FEV_1 (Fig. 3.33) [9, 10].

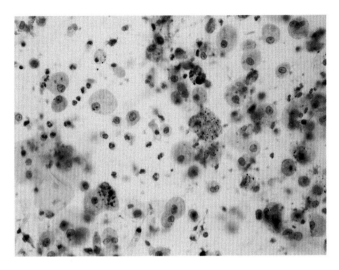

Fig. 3.33 BAL fluid demonstrates neutrophilia (Papanicolaou [PAP] stain) (Courtesy of Dr. Stephanie Yang)

3.4   Antibody-Mediated Rejection

The diagnosis of antibody-mediated rejection (AMR) of the lung allograft is a controversial area that has not been fully elucidated. In contrast, the diagnosis of AMR has been well defined and described in heart and kidney transplants for several years. In patients with these transplanted organs, it was discovered that the presence of donor-specific antibodies (DSAs) and concurrent capillary inflammation correlated with graft dysfunction and decreased overall graft survival [11, 12]. Investigators also discovered a strong correlation between capillary deposition of a specific complement component, C4d, and the presence of DSAs and graft dysfunction/deterioration [13]. This led to the use of staining for C4d in capillaries as a reliable and specific marker for AMR in these transplant organs. However, investigators looking at these same features in the lung allograft, capillary inflammation and capillary C4d deposition, have found varying results with respect to association with AMR. This is likely due to many factors, including difficulty in evaluating capillaries in small and crushed transbronchial biopsies. Studies that have looked at C4d deposition have found extensive nonspecific staining, and there appear to be very few cases that demonstrate diffuse and strong C4d deposition in the clinical setting of suspected AMR [14–16]. Nevertheless, some studies have found diffuse C4d staining of alveolar capillaries is very suspicious for AMR, but this finding is rare and probably insensitive [17, 18].

Some studies have found a positive and statistically significant association between DSAs and capillary inflammation, arteritis, and/or acute lung injury [4, 19, 20]. Capillary inflammation has been defined as a spectrum ranging from capillary neutrophils above baseline to frank capillaritis with fibrinoid necrosis, alveolar hemorrhage, and karyorrhectic debris. We suggest using the term "capillaritis" only when these severe features are present but noting capillary inflammation with neutrophilia when there are capillary neutrophils above baseline levels. Arteritis suspicious for AMR is endotheliitis in arteries with the absence of perivascular infiltrates. Acute lung injury is a spectrum of changes from interstitial edema with reactive pneumocytes to frank hyaline membranes characteristic of diffuse alveolar damage. When these findings are noted on a biopsy, a clinical search for features of AMR can be suggested, but all of these features are nonspecific and can frequently be seen in the setting of infection or in the immediate post-transplant period. Therefore, thorough clinical investigation, including evaluation of microbiology and serological studies for DSAs, is necessary before the diagnosis of AMR should be considered (Figs. 3.34, 3.35, 3.36, 3.37, and 3.38).

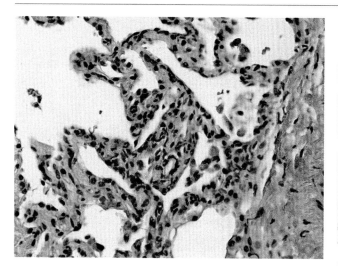

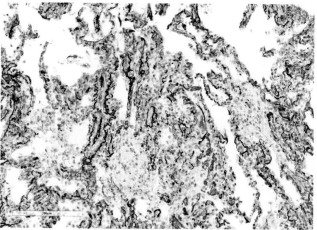

Fig. 3.34 Transbronchial biopsy with focally intense capillary neutrophilia. Note the neutrophils are entirely within capillaries with no involvement of the alveolar space; this is the opposite of what to expect in acute pneumonia. The capillary neutrophilia is a nonspecific finding but should prompt a clinical evaluation to exclude AMR if the patient has no evidence of an infection

Fig. 3.36 C4d immunostain of biopsy from Fig. 3.35. Note the diffuse capillary staining within alveolar walls. Also, note the nonspecific staining of fibrin and elastic tissue. It can be very difficult to determine what structures are staining, leading to interpretation difficulties. Furthermore, many pathologists have noted this diffuse pattern of staining is very infrequently experienced in practice. Therefore, the C4d immunoperoxidase stain is probably an insensitive method for detecting AMR and the stain should be used judiciously (C4d immunoperoxidase stain)

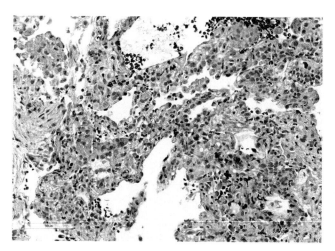

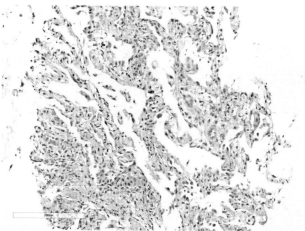

Fig. 3.35 Transbronchial biopsy with capillary inflammation and more pronounced alveolar wall interstitial edema. Note the near absence of inflammatory cells in the alveolar space. This patient had DSAs and clinical evidence of AMR

Fig. 3.37 Transbronchial biopsy with acute lung injury and interstitial edema. Note the scattered inflammatory cells including neutrophils within the interstitium. In the absence of a known etiology, this finding should prompt clinical investigation for AMR

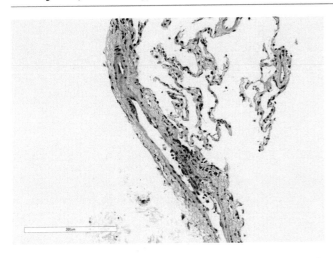

Fig. 3.38 Small arteriole with endotheliitis. This finding is seen in grade A2 rejection, but should also prompt clinical investigation for AMR

3.5 Infections

Lung transplant patients are at increased risk for numerous infections throughout the entire life of the allograft owing to both lifelong antirejection immunosuppression and diminishment of normal defense mechanisms as a consequence of the transplant procedure, including reduced cough reflex and mucociliary clearance [21, 22]. Various infections are relatively more frequent at different times depending on the age of the allograft. Early in the immediate post-transplant period, bacterial infections are overwhelmingly the most common cause of infection. After the patient returns to the community, typical community pathogens are encountered at higher rates in lung transplant patients, and atypical infections, such fungal or more virulent viral infections, may be encountered. Certain infections, including CMV and *Pseudomonas*, have been implicated in the development of BOS in some patients. For this reason, lung transplant patients are carefully clinically monitored for evidence of infection. Pathologically, special stains for organisms may help identify organisms but are generally only indicated if there is a clinical concern or histological features for infection. In our experience, performing organism stains on all lung transplant biopsies is very inefficient (Figs. 3.39, 3.40, 3.41, 3.42, and 3.43).

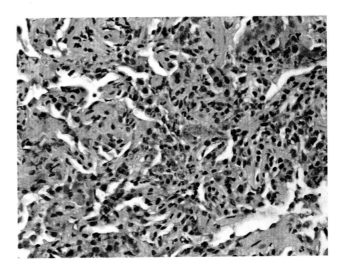

Fig. 3.39 Acute pneumonia. In this case, the alveolar sacs are obscured by acute inflammation including numerous neutrophils. Contrast this with the capillary inflammation seen in Figs. 3.34 and 3.35

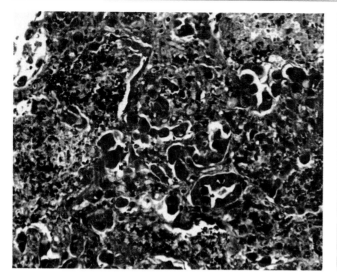

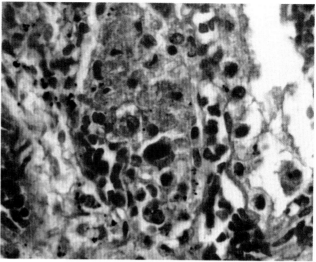

Fig. 3.40 Hemorrhagic alveolar tissue with florid viral inclusions in pneumocyte nuclei and smudgy cytoplasmic expansion. In some nuclei, there are clear "halos" around the inclusion. This is very characteristic of a bona fide viral inclusion. Immunohistochemistry stains or in situ hybridization labeling is necessary to determine viral type. This case demonstrated CMV; most cases of CMV infection will not have such florid lung injury and hemorrhage

Fig. 3.42 Hemorrhagic alveolar tissue with nuclear viral inclusion in the center of the picture from the autopsy of a lung transplant patient

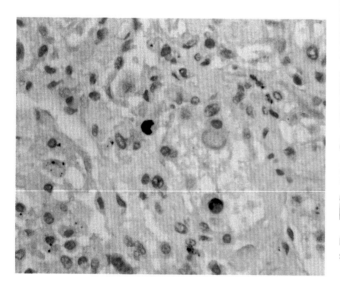

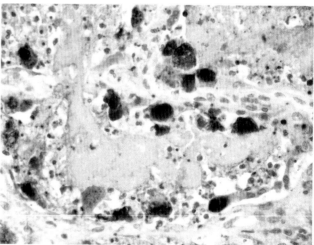

Fig. 3.43 Adenovirus stain of specimen from Fig. 3.42 (Adenovirus stain)

Fig. 3.41 CMV immunostain. Note the distinctive staining of the nuclear inclusion. CMV may also demonstrate cytoplasmic inclusions (not seen on this stain) (CMV stain)

3.6 Other Findings

3.6.1 Ischemia-Reperfusion Injury

The ischemia followed by blood reperfusion encountered by allograft lungs during the transplantation procedure is traumatic to the organ and invariably results in some degree of acute lung injury. In most cases, the acute lung injury is mild and resolves within the first post-transplant month. In cases of severe acute lung injury, primary graft dysfunction (PGD) may develop. PGD is a clinical syndrome characterized by decreased arterial oxygen partial pressure and development of concurrent chest infiltrates. Patients with PGD have high rates of post-transplant morbidity and mortality. The pathological features of ischemia-reperfusion injury are nonspecific acute lung injury, ranging from mild to diffuse alveolar damage with hyaline membranes in the setting of PGD, without evidence of infection. In most early post-transplant biopsies, the presence of ischemia-reperfusion injury may cause interpretive difficulties in cases with possible concurrent rejection or infection and it is important to follow strict diagnostic criteria when rendering pathologic interpretation (Fig. 3.44) [23].

3.6.2 Acute Lung Injury and Organizing Pneumonia

A common finding in transplant transbronchial biopsies is acute lung injury and the etiology may or may not be apparent on the biopsy. In the absence of a clear etiology, clinical correlation is necessary to determine the significance and etiology. In some cases, the findings may be very focal and discovered on a surveillance biopsy. In this setting, the pathologist and clinician may determine the findings are likely not significant. In other cases, there may be clinical features of allograft dysfunction or injury and etiological discovery is important and usually best determined by the clinical team carefully evaluating all pathological, radiological, serological, and microbiological data. Considerations include ischemia-reperfusion injury, severe acute rejection, acute infection including virus, AMR, aspiration, drug injury, or an idiopathic process. The pathological features range from interstitial edema with reactive pneumocytes to severe acute lung injury with hyaline membranes. As the injury progresses and organizes, polyps of organizing pneumonia develop that may fill alveolar sacs and obstruct small airways. Treatment and prognosis is dependent upon both etiology and severity of disease (Figs. 3.45, 3.46, 3.47, and 3.48).

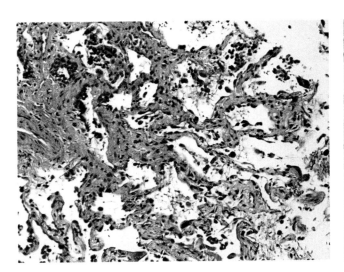

Fig. 3.44 Transbronchial biopsy from a patient 2 weeks post-transplant. There is moderate acute lung injury with interstitial edema, reactive pneumocytes, and collections of discohesive mononuclear cells and denuded respiratory epithelial cells. There is no purulent inflammation to suggest an infectious process. These features are very similar to the reported findings in AMR (Figs. 3.34 to 3.37), but are not suggestive of AMR in the first few weeks after transplant

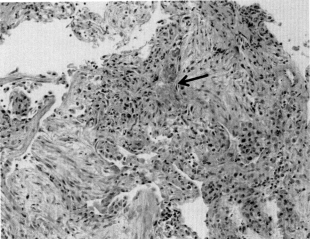

Fig. 3.45 Acute lung injury and florid organizing pneumonia. The fibrin in the center of the picture (*arrow*) along with the scattered inflammatory cells and edema indicate acute lung injury. The polyps of organizing pneumonia are filling most of the airspaces in this image and indicate this process is subacute or organizing

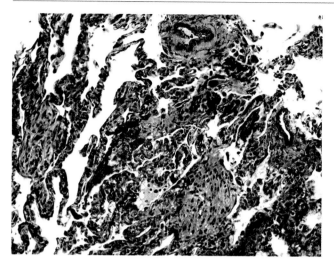

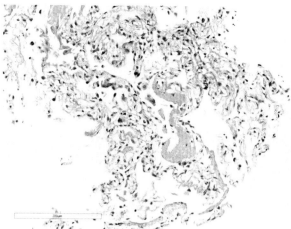

Fig. 3.46 Acute lung injury and organizing pneumonia. The fibrin in this picture is bright red on the trichrome stain. The polyp of organizing pneumonia at the bottom center of this image contains numerous inflammatory cells. The etiology of this process is not evident on this picture (Combined Masson trichrome and elastic van Gieson stain)

Fig. 3.48 Diffuse alveolar damage with hyaline membranes. The hyaline membranes, composed of fibrin and cellular debris, indicate this is severe acute lung injury. The alveolar walls are very edematous and expanded

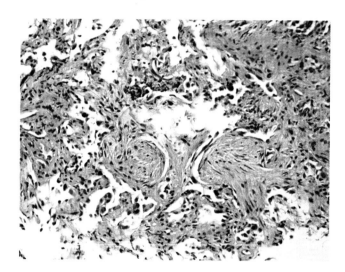

Fig. 3.47 Organizing pneumonia. The etiology of this process is not evident on this picture. Depending on the etiology and clinical context, the polyps may resolve or may contribute to the development of interstitial fibrosis of RAS over time

3.6.3 Aspiration

As discussed previously, lung transplant patients are at increased risk for aspiration due to diminishment of the cough reflex and normal mucociliary clearance mechanisms [1, 22]. Foreign material may be aspirated or may be inadvertently introduced in the lungs during a procedure. The significance depends upon the context, extent, or size of the exogenous material and presence or absence of a concurrent infection. The exogenous material is often polarizable, which can aid in the discovery, and can often be recognized by association with foreign body giant cells (Fig. 3.49).

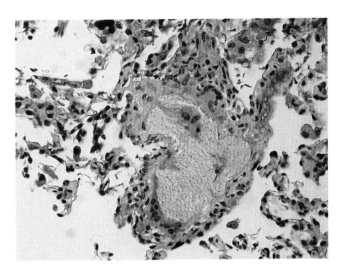

Fig. 3.49 Exogenous foreign material with giant cell reaction. Foreign material can often be highlighted by polarizing the slide. In this case, the substance of the foreign material is unknown

3.6.4 Artifact

Transbronchial lung biopsies are, by their nature, fraught with potential for artifactual distortion and interpretive difficulties. The lung is primarily composed of airspaces and thin-walled alveoli that are easily crushed and distorted during the biopsy procedure. In areas of marked distortion, we tend to refrain from making specific diagnoses if histological structures and anatomical landmarks cannot be identified. Exceptions to this rule include the discovery organisms, foreign material or neoplastic cells. Gently shaking the formalin container with the biopsy material after the procedure may open the airspaces and improve the quality of the histological evaluation (Figs. 3.50 and 3.51).

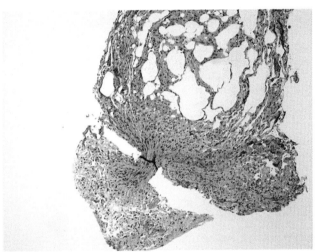

Fig. 3.50 Transbronchial biopsy forceps pinch artifact. In areas of alveolar collapse, we recommend to refrain from making specific diagnoses if the anatomical structures cannot be identified

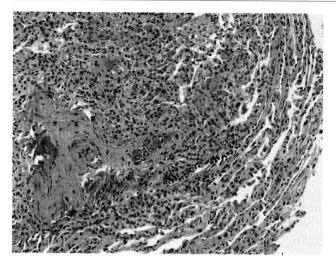

Fig. 3.51 Collapse artifact. There appears to be a vessel with a collection of inflammatory cells within or near it. In the upper portion of the picture, there are relatively frequent neutrophils. However, owing to the collapse artifact, the outline of the vessel appears to be lost and it is not clear where the mononuclear cells are in relation to the vessel or if there is endotheliitis. It is also unclear if the neutrophils are in capillaries, airspaces, areas of procedural hemorrhage, or are at normal baseline level. For all of these reasons, we would not make a firm diagnosis on this image but would examine serial sections or special connective tissue stains to better illustrate the process

3.6.5 Recurrent Disease in the Lung Allograft

Recurrence of disease in the lung allograft is unusual and rarely discovered on the transbronchial biopsy. Sarcoidosis, neoplasms, lymphangioleiomyomatosis (LAM), pulmonary Langerhans cell histiocytosis (PLCH), pulmonary veno-occlusive disease/pulmonary capillary hemangiomatosis (PVOD/PCH), and disease of environmental exposure have all been reported to recur [24–27]. Sarcoidosis is the most common disease to recur in the lung transplant and recurs in 10 % of cases.

3.6.6 Post-transplant Lymphoproliferative Disorder

Lung transplant patients are at the highest risk of solid organ transplant recipients for the development of post-transplant lymphoproliferative disorder (PTLD) which occurs in 6 % of patients [28]. Nevertheless, PTLD is rarely encountered on a transbronchial biopsy. See Chap. 9 for more information.

References

1. Duarte AG, Myers AC. Cough reflex in lung transplant recipients. Lung. 2012;190:23–7.
2. Stewart S, Fishbein MC, Snell GI, Berry GJ, Boehler A, Burke MM, et al. Revision of the 1996 Working Formulation for the Standardization of Nomenclature in the Diagnosis of Lung Rejection. J Heart Lung Transplant. 2007;26:1229–42.
3. Yousem SA, Berry GJ, Cagle PT, Chamberlain D, Husain AN, Hruban RH, et al. Revision of the 1990 Working Formulation for the Classification of Pulmonary Allograft Rejection: Lung Rejection Study Group. J Heart Lung Transplant. 1996;15: 1–15.
4. Wallace WD, Weigt SS, Farver CF. Update on pathology of antibody-mediated rejection in the lung allograft. Curr Opin Organ Transplant. 2014;19:303–8.
5. Verleden GM, Raghu G, Meyer KC, Glanville AR, Corris P. A new classification system for chronic lung allograft dysfunction. J Heart Lung Transplant. 2014;33(2):127–33.
6. Ahmad U, Wang Z, Bryant AS, Kim AW, Kukreja J, Mason DP, et al. Outcomes for lung transplantation for lung cancer in the United Network for Organ Sharing Registry. Ann Thorac Surg. 2012;94:935–40; discussion 940–1.
7. Saggar R, Ross DJ, Saggar R, Zisman DA, Gregson A, Lynch III JP, et al. Pulmonary hypertension associated with lung transplantation obliterative bronchiolitis and vascular remodeling of the allograft. Am J Transplant. 2008;8:1921–30.
8. Sato M, Waddell TK, Wagnetz U, Roberts HC, Hwang DM, Haroon A, et al. Restrictive allograft syndrome (RAS): a novel form of chronic lung allograft dysfunction. J Heart Lung Transplant. 2011;30:735–42.
9. Verleden SE, Vandermeulen E, Ruttens D, Vos R, Vaneylen A, Dupont LJ, et al. Neutrophilic reversible allograft dysfunction (NRAD) and restrictive allograft syndrome (RAS). Semin Respir Crit Care Med. 2013;34:352–60.
10. de Jong PA, Vos R, Verleden GM, Vanaudenaerde BM, Verschakelen JA. Thin-section computed tomography findings before and after azithromycin treatment of neutrophilic reversible lung allograft dysfunction. Eur Radiol. 2011;21:2466–74.
11. Mauiyyedi S, Colvin RB. Humoral rejection in kidney transplantation: new concepts in diagnosis and treatment. Curr Opin Nephrol Hypertens. 2002;11:609–18.
12. Stewart S, Winters GL, Fishbein MC, Tazelaar HD, Kobashigawa J, Abrams J, et al. Revision of the 1990 Working Formulation for the Standardization of Nomenclature in the Diagnosis of Heart Rejection. J Heart Lung Transplant. 2005; 24:1710–20.
13. Feucht HE. Complement C4d in graft capillaries—the missing link in the recognition of humoral alloreactivity. Am J Transplant. 2003;3:646–52.
14. Wallace WD, Reed EF, Ross D, Lassman CR, Fishbein MC. C4d staining of pulmonary allograft biopsies: an immunoperoxidase study. J Heart Lung Transplant. 2005;24:1565–70.
15. Magro CM, Deng A, Pope-Harman A, Waldman WJ, Bernard Collins A, Adams PW, et al. Humorally mediated posttransplantation septal capillary injury syndrome as a common form of pulmonary allograft rejection: a hypothesis. Transplantation. 2002;74:1273–80.
16. Westall GP, Snell GI, McLean C, Kotsimbos T, Williams T, Magro C. C3d and C4d deposition early after lung transplantation. J Heart Lung Transplant. 2008;27:722–8.
17. Berry G, Burke M, Andersen C, Angelini A, Bruneval P, Calabrese F, et al. Pathology of pulmonary antibody-mediated rejection: 2012 update from the Pathology Council of the ISHLT. J Heart Lung Transplant. 2013;32:14–21.
18. Yousem SA, Zeevi A. The histopathology of lung allograft dysfunction associated with the development of donor-specific HLA alloantibodies. Am J Surg Pathol. 2012;36:987–92.
19. Astor TL, Galantowicz M, Phillips A, Palafox J, Baker P. Pulmonary capillaritis as a manifestation of acute humoral allograft rejection following infant lung transplantation. Am J Transplant. 2009;9:409–12.
20. DeNicola MM, Weigt SS, Belperio JA, Reed EF, Ross DJ, Wallace WD. Pathologic findings in lung allografts with anti-HLA antibodies. J Heart Lung Transplant. 2013;32:326–32.
21. Stewart S. Pulmonary infections in transplantation pathology. Arch Pathol Lab Med. 2007;131:1219–31.
22. Hafkin J, Blumberg E. Infections in lung transplantation: new insights. Curr Opin Organ Transplant. 2009;14:483–7.
23. Lee JC, Christie JD. Primary Graft Dysfunction. Proc Am Thorac Soc. 2009;6:39–46.
24. Shah L. Lung transplantation in sarcoidosis. Semin Respir Crit Care Med. 2007;28:134–40.
25. Nine JS, Yousem SA, Paradis IL, Keenan R, Griffith BP. Lymphangioleiomyomatosis: recurrence after lung transplantation. J Heart Lung Transplant. 1994;13:714–9.
26. Dauriat G, Mal H, Thabut G, Mornex JF, Bertocchi M, Tronc F, et al. Lung transplantation for pulmonary Langerhans' cell histiocytosis: a multicenter analysis. Transplantation. 2006;81:746–50.
27. Lee C, Suh RD, Krishnam MS, Lai CK, Fishbein MC, Wallace WD, et al. Recurrent pulmonary capillary hemangiomatosis after bilateral lung transplantation. J Thorac Imaging. 2010;25:W89–92.
28. Reams BD, McAdams HP, Howell DN, Steele MP, Davis RD, Palmer SM. Posttransplant lymphoproliferative disorder: incidence, presentation, and response to treatment in lung transplant recipients. Chest. 2003;124:1242–9.

Kidney Transplant Pathology

4

M. Fernando Palma-Diaz and Jonathan E. Zuckerman

Renal allograft biopsies are the gold standard for evaluation of allograft dysfunction owing to their high diagnostic and prognostic value, thus dramatically affecting treatment decisions. Graft dysfunction is reported to occur in 30 % of recipients in the first year following transplant [1]. Subsequent rates decline to 2–4 % per year. Allograft biopsy interpretations result in changes to the clinical diagnosis in 36 % of cases [2].

Kidney transplant biopsies are performed to investigate the cause of allograft dysfunction ("indication biopsy"), at predefined intervals ("protocol biopsy"), at the time of implantation ("time-zero biopsy") and to evaluate transplant suitability. Indication biopsies are obtained to evaluate for cause of graft dysfunction including rejection, acute tubular injury, recurrent renal disease, infectious processes, and drug toxicity; and to determine the extent of tubulointerstitial scarring. The biopsy interpretation can be challenging because several disease processes may occur simultaneously. Furthermore, pathological evaluation is often time-sensitive because treatment decisions depend on the results and preliminary impressions often need to be rendered before all studies on a biopsy are complete.

4.1 Technical Considerations

4.1.1 Specimen Adequacy

An adequate sample is imperative for proper evaluation of the renal allograft. Adequate core biopsies should contain at least 10 glomeruli and 2 arterial segments, although biopsies with 7–10 glomeruli and 1 artery are considered marginally adequate. Biopsies with fewer than 7 glomeruli and without arteries are suboptimal for evaluation of rejection or recurrent disease or assessment of chronicity. In addition, it is also recommended that two separate core biopsies be obtained whenever possible to increase the diagnostic yield of the sample because rejection can be focal in the early stages [3]. The diameter of the needle is an important consideration because 16-gauge needles provide more diagnostically adequate tissue without an increase in the complication rate compared with 18-gauge needles according to one large study [4]. It is important to bear in mind that a few diagnoses can be made in samples composed of medulla only, the most important being polyomavirus nephropathy (PVN). At UCLA, histotechnologists evaluate the adequacy of allograft (and native) kidney biopsies immediately after sampling. Evaluation is performed using a stereotactic microscope to facilitate identification of glomeruli, which can be seen as red circles or bulging hemispheres on the tissue core (Fig. 4.1). Adequacy is communicated directly to the clinician performing the biopsy; additional biopsy material can be immediately collected if needed. The tissue core is subsequently divided into three containers intended for the different diagnostic modalities used in the evaluation of renal transplant biopsies, as each requires a different fixative. For light microscopy (LM), 10 % neutral buffered formalin is the most commonly used medium because of its wide availability and ease of use. Bouin fixative is a suitable alternative, with the major drawback being decreased effectiveness for immunoperoxidase and in situ hybridization studies. Samples intended for immunofluorescence microscopy (IF) can be snap frozen or placed in Michel's transport media or Zeus

M.F. Palma-Diaz, MD (✉) • J.E. Zuckerman, MD, PhD
Department of Pathology and Laboratory Medicine,
David Geffen School of Medicine at the University of California,
Los Angeles, Los Angeles, CA, USA
e-mail: fpalmadiaz@mednet.ucla.edu

© Springer International Publishing Switzerland 2016
W.D. Wallace, B.V. Naini (eds.), *Practical Atlas of Transplant Pathology*, DOI 10.1007/978-3-319-23054-2_4

fixative. Both Michel's and Zeus solutions offer antigen preservation comparable with that of snap freezing but allow storage and transport of tissue at room temperature for up to 72 h. For electron microscopy (EM), gluteraldehyde and the gluteraldehyde-based Karnovsky's fixative provide rapid stabilization of proteins by cross-linking, thus making these fixatives ideal for this use. As a general rule, the majority of the cortical sample should be submitted for LM because it provides the highest diagnostic yield in most transplant cases. Moreover, IF and EM require only a few glomeruli and, in certain circumstances (see later), EM can be skipped altogether.

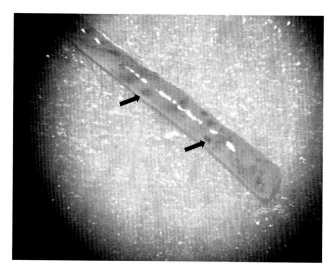

Fig. 4.1 Renal tissue core obtained with a 16-gauge needle contains several blood-filled glomeruli, which appear as congested bulging hemispheres (*arrows*). Sclerotic and inflamed glomeruli with little or no circulating blood are notoriously difficult to identify. Medullary tissue (*not shown*) is easy to recognize because it displays streaks or parallel lines corresponding to tubules and has no glomeruli

4.1.2 Specimen Processing

4.1.2.1 Light Microscopy

The Banff 97 recommendation [3] for specimen processing is as follows: at least seven slides with multiple sequential 3- to 4-μm sections should be cut. Three of these slides should be stained with hematoxylin and eosin (H&E) stain, three with periodic acid–Schiff (PAS) stain or silver stains, and one with a trichrome stain. At UCLA, eight sequential sections of 3-μm thickness are cut. Levels 1–4 are stained sequentially as follows: H&E, trichrome, PAS, and Jones methenamine silver (JMS) stain. Levels 5–8 are stained in a similar fashion. The turnaround time for these studies is usually less than 24 h from time of biopsy. We routinely process H&E-stained sections for same-day analysis when clinically indicated. For STAT cases, H&E-stained slides can be obtained within 4 h, thus allowing for preliminary evaluation of acute cellular rejection, acute tubular injury/necrosis (ATI/ATN), the presence or absence of thrombosis, and estimation of tubulointerstitial scarring. For more detailed assessment, special stains are needed.

4.1.2.2 Immunofluorescence Microscopy

The primary role of IF in the evaluation of the renal transplant is to assess for C4d deposition in antibody-mediated rejection (AMR). Therefore, C4d immunofluorescence studies are required in every case. In addition, IF studies are helpful in identification of recurrent and de novo glomerular disease. IF has little role in the diagnosis of T-cell–mediated rejection except to rule out other differential diagnoses. A full IF panel (including immunoglobulin G [IgG], IgA, IgM, C3, C1q, fibrinogen, and kappa and lambda light chains) is generally required only on samples where glomerular disease is suspected. On all transplant cases, the minimal IF panel for our group includes C4d and fibrinogen (to aid in the assessment of thrombotic microangiopathy—discussed later).

4.1.2.3 Electron Microscopy

Gluteraldehyde-fixed tissue is embedded into epoxy resin and 1-μm sections are cut. Survey ("thick") sections are stained with toluidine blue to evaluate the tissue and assess for the presence of glomeruli by LM prior to EM analysis. In some cases, these sections may contain diagnostic material not otherwise seen in the tissue for LM. Like IF, EM has a more limited role in the transplant biopsy compared with native kidney biopsies. EM is most useful for evaluating features of chronic antibody-mediated rejection (CAMR; see later) and cases with suspected recurrent or de novo glomerular disease. EM is of no practical use in the diagnosis of T-cell–mediated rejection. EM need not be performed on every biopsy. In general, EM should be performed when glomerular disease is suspected. At UCLA, we perform EM in every new transplant case, in patients without prior biopsies over the past 6 months, and as clinically or pathologically indicated.

4.2 Pathological Classification of Diseases of the Renal Allograft and the Banff Classification

Renal allografts are targets for (1) alloreactive immune response (rejection) including T-cell–mediated rejection and AMR; (2) pathology related to the transplant procedure such as ATI/ATN due to prolonged ischemia time, vessel thrombosis, and ureteral obstruction; (3) medication-induced toxicity or disease susceptibility (immunosuppression) including calcineurin inhibitor (CNI) toxicity, PVN, and post-transplant lymphoproliferative disorder (PTLD); and (4) diseases that affect native kidneys, which may represent recurrent or de novo disease.

The differential diagnosis for allograft dysfunction changes over time. Within the first 6 months of transplantation (particularly <3 months), the primary differential diagnosis of allograft dysfunction includes acute rejection, acute ischemic injury, acute CNI toxicity, and acute pyelonephritis.

In allografts greater than 6 months old, the primary differential diagnosis of dysfunction includes CAMR, chronic CNI toxicity, hypertension, chronic obstruction/reflux nephropathy, chronic pyelonephritis, PVN, glomerular disease (recurrent or de novo), PTLD, and chronic changes of unclear etiology.

4.2.1 Banff Criteria

The most widely used scheme for the grading and reporting of kidney transplant pathology is the Banff classification [5]. Since its inception in 1993, the classification system has been continually revised and is still being refined [5]. The use of Banff criteria in grading kidney transplant rejection allows a measure of standardization for the improvement of diagnostic consensus, publication, and research. Furthermore, the Banff grading is based primarily on LM features that can be identified and graded and subsequently synthesized into a classification of rejection. The Banff classification uses six major diagnostic categories for renal allograft biopsies (Table 4.1) [6].

Table 4.1 Banff renal allograft diagnostic categories [6]

1. Normal	No allograft pathology
2. Antibody-mediated changes	Owing to documentation of circulating anti-DSAs, and C4d, or allograft pathology (may coincide with categories 3, 4, 5, and 6)
3. Borderline changes	Suspicious for acute T-cell–mediated rejection (may coincide with categories 2, 5, and 6)
4. T-cell–mediated rejection	May coincide with categories 2, 5, and 6
5. sInterstitial fibrosis and TA	No evidence of any specific etiology
6. Other	Changes not considered to be due to rejection, acute or chronic, may include isolated g, cg, or cv lesions (may coincide with categories 2, 3, 4, and 5)

Cg chronic glomerulopathy score, *cv* vascular fibrous intimal thickening score, *g* glomerulitis score

4.3 Acute Allograft Rejection

4.3.1 Acute T-Cell–Mediated Rejection

4.3.1.1 Clinical Presentation

Acute T-cell–mediated rejection (acute cellular rejection [ACR]) is most common in the first few months following transplant; however, it can occur at any time post transplant [7]. Severe ACR classically presents as an acute increase in creatinine with decreased urine output, weight gain, fever, and graft tenderness and swelling. Low-grade ACR can be clinically silent and appear as "smoldering ACR" on a protocol biopsy. However, there is great variability in the clinical presentations of all grades of ACR. Hematuria and proteinuria are uncommon manifestations of ACR.

4.3.1.2 Microscopic Features

The most common morphological features of ACR are interstitial inflammation and tubulitis. In severe cases, endarteritis may be observed.

Interstitium T-cells and macrophages are the predominant cells in the infiltrate, but variable numbers of plasma cells, neutrophils, and eosinophils may also be seen. Interstitial edema is an accompanying feature in the great majority of cases (Fig. 4.2). The inflammation is cortical and patchy; however, in severe cases, spillover into the medulla can be seen. Occasional, marked plasma cell accumulation is observed—so-called "plasma cell–rich" ACR (Fig. 4.3). The differential diagnosis for plasma cell–rich infiltrates in a renal allograft includes PVN and post-transplant lymphoproliferative disorder (PTLD); therefore, these considerations need to be ruled out. Prominent neutrophilic infiltration should raise suspicion for acute AMR, particularly if neutrophils are within peritubular capillaries (PTCs), or acute pyelonephritis, if accompanied by neutrophil casts in tubules (Fig. 4.4).

The Banff score for interstitial inflammation (i) is based on percentage involvement of nonscarred cortical parenchyma. However, data are emerging suggesting that even inflammation in scarred cortex is significant [8, 9]. Therefore, two interstitial inflammation scoring systems have been proposed: (i) percentage of inflammation in the nonatrophic cortex (Table 4.2) and (ti) total cortical inflammation. In the current classification system, a diagnosis of ACR requires inflammation involving at least 25 % of the nonscarred cortex (i2).

Tubules The key morphological feature of ACR is tubule-infiltrating lymphocytes—tubulitis—which is best appreciated on PAS-stained sections where the tubular basement membrane can be visualized. Tubule-infiltrating lymphocytes appear as small, dark, basally located nuclei compared with the larger, pale, more apically located epithelial cell nuclei (Fig. 4.5). Tubulitis in areas of tubular atrophy (TA) is not currently considered a manifestation of ACR. The Banff tubulitis score (t) is based on number of mononuclear cells per transverse tubule cross section (or per 10 epithelial nuclei in longitudinal cuts) (Table 4.3).

Glomeruli Glomeruli are usually spared in cases of tubulointerstitial ACR. However, glomerulitis, defined as the presence of glomerular intracapillary mononuclear inflammatory cell infiltration and endothelial cell swelling resulting in narrowing/occlusion of at least one capillary lumen, is occasionally observed in cases of ACR in the absence of acute AMR. The glomerulitis of ACR consists of T-cell glomerular infiltrates (versus macrophage infiltrates in AMR) [10]. However, glomerulitis is not included as a criterion of ACR (see Sect. 4.4).

Vessels Vascular rejection may be a manifestation of severe ACR. Morphologically, this form of ACR is characterized by the presence of endarteritis (also known as intimal arteritis or endothelialitis), which predominantly affects arcuate and interlobular caliber arterial vessels, although arterioles may also be involved. The endothelial cells of the affected arteries appear "reactive" with increased basophilic cytoplasm and lifting from the underlying arterial media. The presence of subintimal infiltrating mononuclear inflammatory cells is the key diagnostic feature (Fig. 4.6). A single involved artery is sufficient for the diagnosis. Adherent, luminal mononuclear cells (Fig. 4.7) are not diagnostic of endarteritis, but warrant careful examination—including obtaining additional levels—because this finding is commonly associated with endarteritis. Endarteritis seen only at the biopsy edges should also be interpreted with caution, and in this setting, a diagnosis of suspicious for ACR vascular rejection may be most appropriate. In severe cases of vascular rejection, transmural inflammation and fibrinoid necrosis of arteries is observed. The Banff classification scores arteritis (v) based on the degree of luminal narrowing as a result of endarteritis in the most affected artery (Table 4.4). Arteries showing transmural inflammation and/or fibrinoid necrosis are automatically scored as v3.

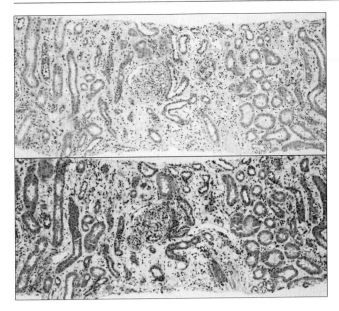

Fig. 4.2 Low-power view of the renal cortex shows diffuse interstitial inflammation associated with marked separation of the tubules as a result of interstitial edema, confirmed with the trichrome stain (*bottom*). Interstitial edema is a common accompanying feature of active interstitial inflammatory processes of any kind, including ACR

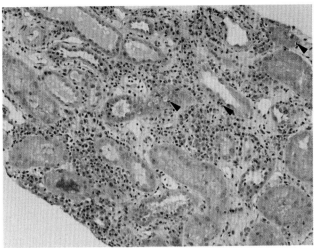

Fig. 4.3 There is a dense infiltrate primarily composed of clusters of plasma cells, associated with several foci of lymphocytic tubulitis (*arrowheads*). The differential diagnosis includes PTLD, PVN, and plasma cell-rich ACR. There are no reliable histological features to distinguish between these possibilities, and therefore, additional work-up with IHC stains is required

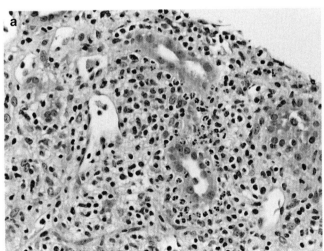

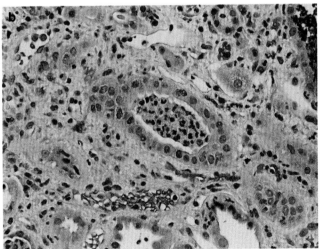

Fig. 4.4 (a) Interstitial inflammation with numerous neutrophils is not a typical feature of ACR and instead should raise suspicion for acute pyelonephritis (H&E, 200×). (b) The presence of intraluminal accumulations of neutrophils (neutrophilic casts) such as this one in a collecting duct represents strong evidence for a diagnosis of acute pyelonephritis and should warrant correlation with urine studies including cultures (H&E; 400×)

Table 4.2 Scoring of interstitial inflammation in nonscarred cortex (i) [3]

Banff score	Percentage of nonscarred cortex inflamed
i0	<10
i1	10–25
i2	26–50
i3	>50

The ti scoring system corresponds to the i system but includes areas of scarring

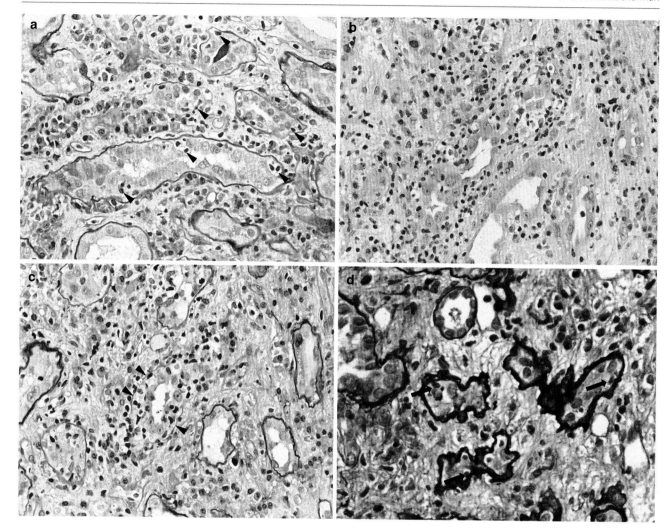

Fig. 4.5 (**a**) Several tubules show foci of tubulitis (*arrowheads*). Lymphocytes are smaller and have a darker nucleus compared with the tubular epithelial cells and often exhibit a "halo." The tubular epithelial cells are displaced apically and exhibit reactive nuclear changes including enlargement and prominent nucleoli. There is an associated inflammatory cell infiltrate in the interstitium that includes activated lymphocytes (lymphoblasts), plasma cells, and monocytes (PAS stain). (**b**) In cases with severe tubulointerstitial ACR, the lymphocytes may obscure tubular structures, making it hard to identify foci of tubulitis.

(**c**) The PAS stain is helpful in highlighting the residual basement membrane (*arrowheads*), thus facilitating visualization of the same tubule. In examples with extensive disruption of basement membranes, focal granulomatous inflammation may occur (*not shown*). (**d**) Atrophic tubules appear shrunken and demonstrate wrinkling and thickening of the basement membranes. Lymphocytic infiltration of atrophic tubules (*arrows*) is nonspecific and not diagnostic of ACR. However, if accompanied by tubulitis in nonscarred tubules, it may be indicative of a subacute cellular rejection process (PAS stain)

Table 4.3 Scoring of tubulitis (t) [3]

Banff score	Mononuclear cells/tubule
t0	0
t1	1–4
t2	5–10
t3	>10

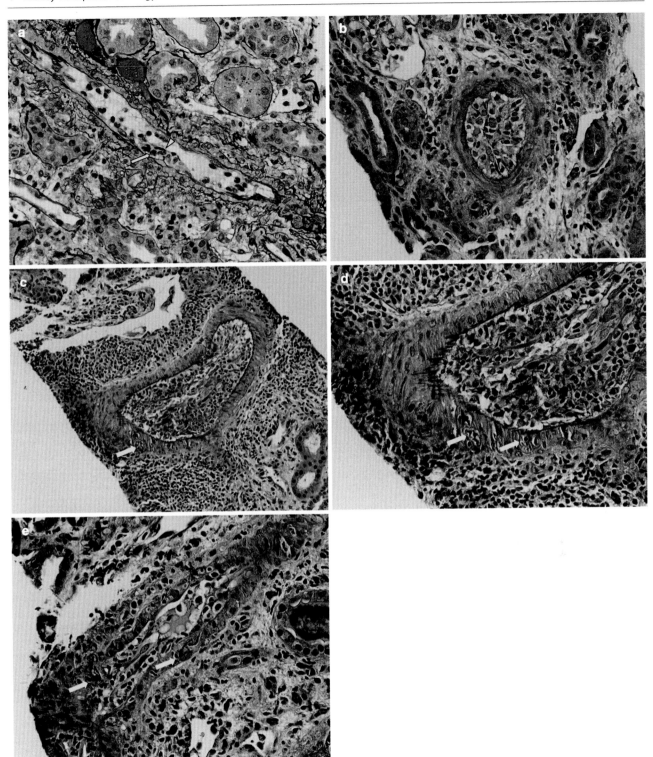

Fig. 4.6 (a) A small artery with endarteritis characterized by focal lymphocytic infiltration of the intima (*arrows*) causing lifting of the overlying endothelial cells (*arrowhead*) and mild narrowing of the lumen (Banff v1 score). The endothelial cells appear plump and prominent and there are several adherent leukocytes in the lumen (Jones methenamine silver stain). (b) A Banff v2 lesion involving a small artery, characterized by severe endarteritis leading to complete luminal occlusion (Trichrome–elastic Van Gieson [EVG] stain). (c) An interlobular artery shows severe endarteritis. In addition, there is focal transmural inflammation (*arrow*), thus categorizing this as a Banff v3 lesion (Trichrome-EVG stain). (d) On higher magnification, lymphocytes are seen infiltrating both the smooth muscle cell layer (*arrows*) and the lumen (Trichrome-EVG stain). (e) An example of fibrinoid necrosis involving the wall of a small artery (Banff v3 lesion). Trichrome stains are particularly useful in recognizing areas of fibrinoid necrosis, which appear as accumulations of bright red granular material corresponding to fibrin (Trichrome stain)

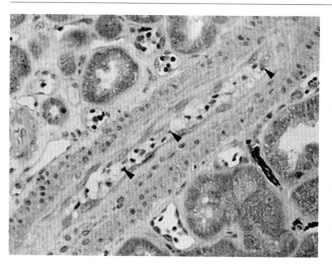

Fig. 4.7 An artery with plump endothelial cells and several margin-ated and adherent leukocytes (*arrowheads*); however, no lymphocytes infiltrating the intima are seen. Although this is not diagnostic of vascu-lar rejection, it should prompt careful search for endarteritis because both typically coexist

4.3.1.3 Immunofluorescence Microscopy

IF is of limited practical use in the diagnosis of ACR. Fibrinoid necrosis is highlighted by staining for fibrinogen. C4d stain-ing of PTCs would indicate concomitant AMR. Focal, granu-lar staining of tubular basement membranes for IgG, C3, and C4d is seen in a small subset of cases of PVN (see later).

4.3.1.4 Classification of ACR

Banff classifies ACR into three grades (Table 4.5). Grade I ACR consists of greater than 25 % interstitial inflammation with moderate or severe tubulitis. Any vascular rejection is automatically classified as at least ACR grade II, regardless of tubulointerstitial inflammation.

Borderline	OR	Any tubulitis (>t0) with <25 % interstitial inflammation ($\leq$i1)
		>25 % interstitial inflammation (i2,i3) with mild tubulitis (t1)

Table 4.4 Scoring of arteritis (v) [3]

Banff score	% of luminal area lost as a result of endarteritis
v0	0
v1	<25
v2	$\geq$25
v3	Transmural inflammation or fibrinoid necrosis

Table 4.5 Classification of ACR [3]

Grade I	>25 % interstitial inflammation (i2, i3)	A	With moderate tubulitis (t2)
		B	With severe tubulitis (t3)
Grade II	Endarteritis	A	Mild to moderate (v1)
		B	Severe (v2)
Grade III	Transmural arteritis or fibrinoid necrosis (v3)		

4.3.1.5 Borderline/Suspicious for ACR

This category is used in cases with tubulointerstitial inflammation or tubulitis that do not meet criteria for a diagnosis of ACR. Borderline changes are observed in approximately 20 % of protocol biopsies 1 year post transplant [11]. Interestingly, there is poor intra- and interobserver reproducibility of this diagnostic category. In addition, management of patients with borderline lesions varies among centers. Besides early rejection, the differential diagnosis for borderline lesions includes other causes of low-level inflammatory cell infiltrate such as ATI/ATN, CNI toxicity, viral infection, and drug-induced hypersensitivity reactions.

4.3.1.6 Treated/Resolving ACR

Resolving/treated ACR is characterized by tubulitis out of proportion to the interstitial inflammation, sometimes associated with early interstitial fibrosis and TA (Fig. 4.8). Correlation with prior biopsies and clinical history is essential for this diagnosis.

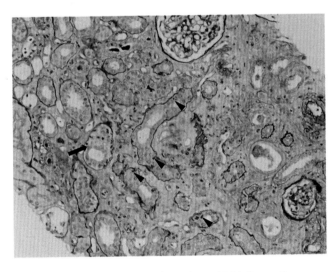

Fig. 4.8 Tubulitis out of proportion to interstitial inflammation sometimes accompanied by mild tubulointerstitial scarring is commonly seen in biopsies from patients who have received treatment for ACR. In this example, there are frequent and prominent foci of tubulitis involving mildly atrophic tubules (*arrowheads*) as well as nonatrophic tubules (*arrow*). There is only a sparse interstitial inflammatory cell infiltrate. This patient had been diagnosed with ACR type IB on the prior biopsy a few weeks earlier and had received immunosuppression treatment (PAS stain)

4.4 Acute Antibody-Mediated Rejection

4.4.1 Clinical Presentation

Occurs in patients who develop de novo donor-specific antibodies (DSAs) after transplant or those patients with preexisting DSAs from presensitization (blood transfusion, pregnancy, prior transplant). Acute antibody-mediated rejection (AAMR) is most common up to 3 weeks post transplantation, but may occur at any time (de novo DSAs usually take approximately 2 weeks to form, so very early AAMR would be due to preformed antibodies). AAMR typically presents with acute oliguric renal failure often requiring dialysis. The overall frequency of AAMR following transplant is 6 %, but it ranges from 8 to 43 % in presensitized patients [12]. One study found that AAMR criteria are met in nearly 24 % of biopsies for acute rejection [13].

4.4.2 Microscopic Features

Morphological manifestations of AAMR include (1) ATI without other apparent cause, (2) capillary inflammation (peritubular capillaritis, glomerulitis), (3) acute thrombotic microangiopathy (TMA), and (4) intimal or transmural arteritis. These may occur alone or in combination.

The histological hallmark of AAMR is microvascular injury in the form of glomerulitis and peritubular capillaritis. PTCs are often dilated and show increased leukocytes, including neutrophils and/or monocytes/macrophages (Fig. 4.9). Glomerulitis is a common finding in AAMR. As with peritubular capillaritis, the leukocytes may consist of mononuclear cells or neutrophils (compared with glomerulitis in ACR, which is T-cell predominant) (Fig. 4.10). Glomeruli may also show features of acute TMA including reactive-appearing endothelial cells, fibrin thrombi, and dissolution of the mesangium (mesangiolysis) (Fig. 4.11).

To be diagnostically significant, peritubular capillaritis has to be present in at least 10 % of the PTCs in the cortex. Banff PTC inflammation grading (ptc score) depends on the average number of intraluminal leukocytes and ranges from ptc0 to ptc3. Areas affected by acute pyelonephritis or necrosis and the subcapsular cortex should not be considered. Caution should also be taken not to score inflammatory cells in the medullary vasa recta. Banff glomerulitis is scored based on the percentage of glomeruli involved from g0 to g3 (Table 4.6).

ATI/ATN is present in 75 % of AAMR biopsies [14]. In our experience, ATI/ATN is too nonspecific to be considered a feature of AAMR, unless it is accompanied by at least mild interstitial inflammation and/or at least minimal peritubular capillaritis. The presence of significant mononuclear tubulitis should be interpreted as concurrent ACR and is reported in 30–80 % of

AAMR biopsies [14, 15]. Very mild tubulitis is a common attendant finding in ATI/ATN and, therefore, should not be regarded as a manifestation of concomitant ACR; however, it can make the distinction from "borderline ACR" difficult.

There are no specific interstitial changes in AAMR. Interstitial edema with minimal/mild mononuclear inflammation (not diagnostic for ACR) may be present in pure AAMR. Interstitial hemorrhage and cortical infarction

may be seen in patients with severe arterial involvement or TMA.

As with ACR, arterial injury in AAMR ranges from mild and limited to the intima (endarteritis) to severe with fibrinoid necrosis and minimal mononuclear cell infiltrate or transmural arteritis. A TMA pattern of vascular injury with mucoid intimal thickening and erythrocyte fragments may be present; however, arterial thrombosis is unusual.

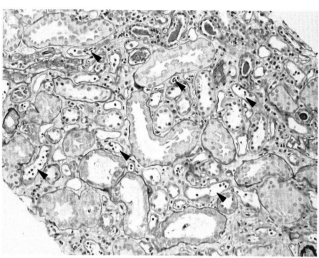
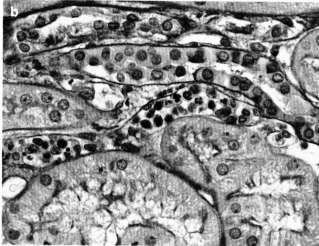

Fig. 4.9 (a) PTCs, best seen in PAS-stained sections, appear distended and contain increased numbers of circulating leukocytes. In the absence of significant interstitial inflammation as in this case, this finding is

more specific for AAMR. (b) In most cases, intracapillary leukocytes comprise a mixed population including mononuclear cells and neutrophils. Occasionally, neutrophils can predominate

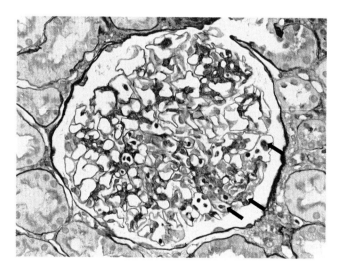

Fig. 4.10 A glomerulus shows intraluminal mononuclear leukocytes associated with endothelial cell swelling in capillary loops in a segmental distribution (arrowheads). Mononuclear infiltrates may represent ACR or AMR. The presence of neutrophils (not shown) would favor AMR over ACR (PAS; 200×)

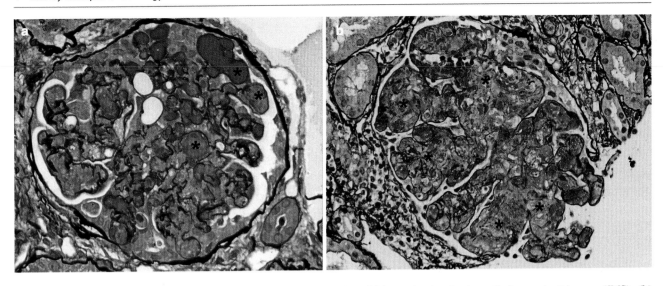

Fig. 4.11 Features of acute TMA are variable, and morphology cannot reliably distinguish among the different causes. In the transplant setting, AAMR and CNI toxicity are the two most common etiologies. (**a**) Fibrin thrombi occluding several glomerular capillary lumens (*asterisks*) can be the dominant finding as in this case (JMS). (**b**) Mesangiolysis or dissolution of the mesangial matrix such as seen in this glomerulus can be another morphological feature of TMA, and it results in a fibrillary appearance of affected mesangial regions (*asterisks*) (JMS)

Table 4.6 Scoring of microvascular inflammation [3, 6]

Glomerulitis (g)		PTCs	
Banff score	% Glomeruli involved	Banff score	Inflammatory cells per capillary
g0	0	ptc0	<10 % involvement
g1	1–25	ptc1	<5
g2	26–50	ptc2	5–10
g3	>50	ptc3	>10

4.4.3   Immunofluorescence Microscopy

The classic hallmark of AMR is C4d deposition in PTCs of the cortex and medulla. The fluorescence should be linear, circumferential, and crisp. C4d staining is often seen in glomeruli and arteries; however, these staining patterns are not specific for AMR but serve as internal controls (Fig. 4.12).

To be diagnostically significant, C4d staining should be at least focal (≥10). Of note, C4d staining can decrease or even disappear after treatment of AMR. C4d can also be detected by immunohistochemistry (IHC), but in general is one-degree less sensitive than IF but offers better visualization of the sample (Table 4.7). This is particularly helpful in cases with extensive tubulointerstitial fibrosis where C4d staining by IF is equivocal or difficult to interpret.

The Banff C4d scoring system is based on the percentage of positive throughout biopsy specimen, cortex, and medulla and ranges from C4d0 (0 % staining) to C4d3 (>50 % staining) (Table 4.7) [6].

Fibrinogen, IgM, C3, and C4d staining may be seen in areas of fibrinoid necrosis.

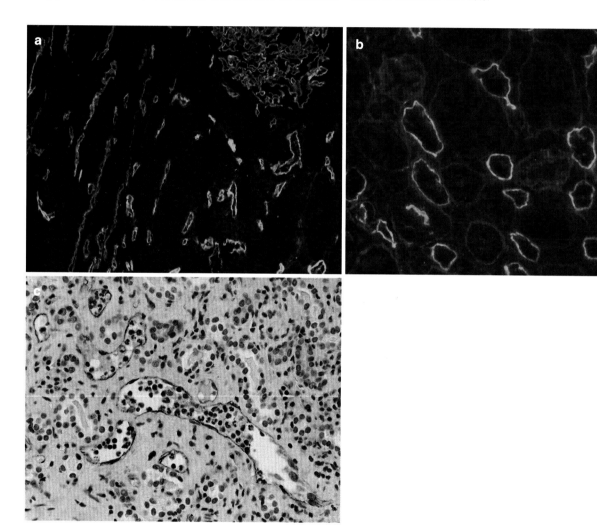

Fig. 4.12 (**a**) This IF image shows C4d staining of both a glomerulus (*upper right corner*) and PTCs. Glomerular and arterial (*not shown*) staining is a ubiquitous phenomenon and does not have clinical significance. Only staining of PTC is a criterion for the diagnosis of AMR. (**b**) C4d staining should be circumferential and strong, as in this example. (**c**) C4d detection by IHC is less sensitive than by IF (*see* Table 4.7), but allows better visualization of the tissue, which is very helpful in cases in which C4d studies by IF are equivocal, such as in biopsies with extensive scarring or necrosis

Table 4.7 Scoring and interpretation of PTC C4d deposition [6]

		% of biopsy (cortex and/or medulla)	Interpretation	
			IF	IHC
C4d0	Negative	0	Negative	Negative
C4d1	Minimal	1–10	Negative	Positive
C4d2	Focal	10–50	Positive	Positive
C4d3	Diffuse	>50	Positive	Positive

4.4.4 Diagnostic Criteria of AAMR

Three major diagnostic criteria must be met for the diagnosis of AAMR (Table 4.8). These are (1) histological evidence of acute tissue injury, (2) evidence of current or recent antibody interaction with vascular endothelium, which may or may not include C4d deposition, and (3) serological evidence of circulating antibodies to DSAs. When only two criteria are met (e.g., negative C4d or no DSAs assay) the findings are interpreted as suspicious for AAMR.

C4d-Negative AMR The diagnosis of AAMR in the absence of C4d staining can be established in two situations: if at least moderate microvascular inflammation is present (i.e., both glomerulitis and peritubular capillaritis) or if increased expression of endothelial activation and injury transcript (ENDATs) or other gene expression markers of endothelial cell injury in biopsy tissue and other AAMR criteria are met, specifically the presence of DSAs [16].

C4d Staining Without Evidence of Rejection Cases with positive C4d staining and lack of morphological findings of acute or chronic rejection may be encountered. This constellation of features is more commonly seen in biopsies from ABO-incompatible allografts, in which it does not appear to result in injury of the graft and, therefore, may represent accommodation [17]. In human leukocyte antigen (HLA)–incompatible allografts, the significance of these findings is uncertain, but at least one study has shown that these may result in development of chronic AMR [18]. For more information, see Chap. 1.

Table 4.8 Banff criteria for AAMR [16]

1. Histological evidence of acute tissue injury (at least one or more)	Microvascular inflammation (ptc > 0 and/or g > 0)
	Intimal or transmural arteritis (v > 0)
	Acute TMA
	Acute tubular injury
2. Evidence of current or recent antibody interaction with vascular endothelium (at least one or more)	ptc C4d staining (C4d2, C4d3 on IF or C4d > 0 on IHC)
	At least moderate microvascular inflammation (g + ptc > 2)
	Increased expression of ENDATs or other gene expression markers of endothelial injury in biopsy tissue
3. Serological evidence of DSAs	HLA, ABO, or other antigens

Diagnosis requires fulfillment of all three criteria. Two criteria fulfillment is considered suspicious for AMR

4.5 Hyperacute AMR

4.5.1 Clinical Presentation

Hyperacute rejection is a rare variant of AAMR (0.1 % of transplants) that results from the presence of preformed anti-DSAs that result in immediate rejection upon transplantation [19]. Its occurrence has largely been eliminated owing to effective cross-match screening. Clinically, it presents within 60 min of transplantation with anuria, high fever, and no perfusion on renal scan; in some cases, it can be noticed by the transplant surgeon when the allograft becomes cyanotic and appears mottled.

4.5.2 Microscopic Features

The microscopic features are those of severe AAMR including interstitial edema and hemorrhage, intravascular coagulation, and cortical necrosis. Arteries show neutrophil infiltration, fibrin thrombi, and fibrinoid necrosis (Fig. 4.13).

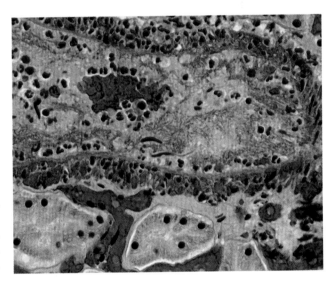

Fig. 4.13 Interlobular artery with organizing thrombus and transmural inflammation with necrosis of the muscular media. These features, especially neutrophilic infiltration through the arterial wall, in the setting of very early graft failure is consistent with hyperacute AMR

4.6   Nonalloimmune Injury

4.6.1   Acute Tubular Injury/Acute Tubular Necrosis

4.6.1.1   Clinical

ATI is a common occurrence in kidney transplant patients and occurs more frequently than in the general healthy population owing to exposure to nephrotoxic drugs and diminished ability to correct fluid imbalances in the renal transplant patient. Therefore, ATN is the first consideration in the differential diagnosis in most patients undergoing kidney biopsy to rule out rejection.

4.6.1.2   Morphological Features

Proximal tubule brush border attenuation with epithelial layer thinning resulting in apparent luminal dilation and non-isometric vacuolization are common early findings. Tubular epithelial cell nuclei may appear activated (prominent nucleoli and vesicular chromatin), and mitoses may be conspicuous. In severe cases, denudation of the epithelial lining into the tubule lumen may occur. In mild cases, a single tubular epithelial cell mitosis is sufficient evidence to support the diagnosis of ATN (Fig. 4.14).

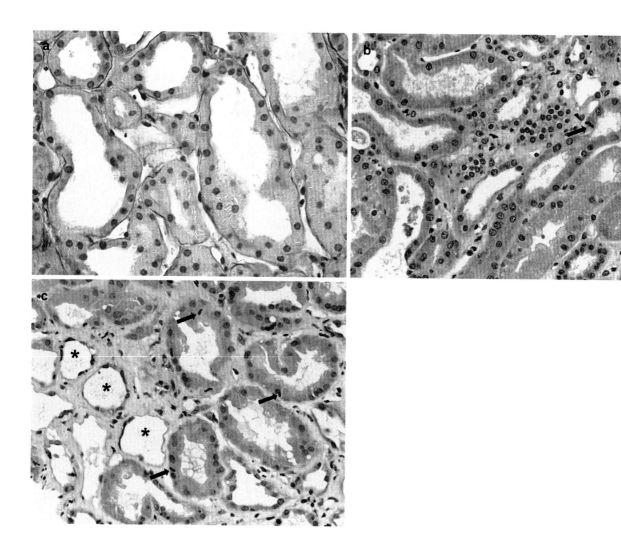

Fig. 4.14 (**a**) In cases of ATI/ATN due to ischemic injury, the proximal tubules are universally involved. Early changes include loss of brush borders resulting in attenuation of the epithelial lining and apparent dilation of the tubular lumens (PAS stain). (**b**) A mitotic figure can be seen (*arrow*). (**c**) With more severe or sustained injury, sloughing of epithelial cells occurs, resulting in empty-appearing tubules with denuded basement membranes (*asterisks*). Reactive nuclear changes include striking reparative changes with nuclear enlargement and prominent nucleoli. In cases with severe nuclear reactive changes, viral infections, particularly PVN, should be considered in the differential diagnosis. In these instances, immunostains to rule out viral infections are helpful. Note adjacent tubules with rare foci of tubulitis (*arrows*), a common accompanying finding in biopsies with severe ATI/ATN, which may make it difficult to distinguish from borderline changes for ACR

4.6.1.3 Differential Diagnosis

This pattern of injury is nonspecific. The primary differential diagnosis includes ischemic injury, acute drug/toxic injury (e.g., CNI toxicity), and AMR (if accompanied by sparse inflammation and other features of AMR). In the absence of other acute diagnostic features, a diagnosis of ATN can be rendered. In our practice, we do not include ATN in the final diagnosis in the presence of other acute findings unless it is severe and appears to be unrelated to the other process.

4.7   Drug Toxicity

4.7.1   CNI Toxicity

4.7.1.1 Clinical

There are two widely used CNIs, cyclosporine and tacrolimus. Although structurally dissimilar, their therapeutic action and toxicity profiles, including histopathological lesions, are similar. Toxicity is dose related.

4.7.1.2 Microscopic Features

CNI toxicity has two major forms: (1) functional and (2) structural [20]. Functional CNI toxicity results from the vasoconstrictive effects of CNIs. There may be no typical morphological changes present in the biopsy. ATI/ATN can be seen; however, functional CNI toxicity is a diagnosis of exclusion. Structural CNI toxicity refers to changes in tubular epithelial cells or vessels induced by CNIs. It is important to keep in mind that few of these changes are specific and the diagnosis of CNI toxicity should be made in the appropriate clinical context. CNI toxicity is divided into early and late stages; however, late-stage changes can develop within weeks of treatment initiation.

Within glomeruli, early CNI toxicity can induce a TMA pattern of injury including endothelial cell swelling, capillary thrombosis, and mesangiolysis (Fig. 4.11). The late glomerular lesion of CNI toxicity—CNI glomerulopathy—results from chronic endothelial cell injury. The morphological picture is that of glomerular basement membrane (GBM) duplication with mild mesangial matrix expansion (similar to transplant glomerulopathy [TG]) (see later). Occasional intracapillary mononuclear cells may be present, but true glomerulitis or endocapillary hypercellularity should raise the possibility of rejection or recurrent/de novo glomerular disease. Ischemic glomerulopathy, with globally wrinkled capillary walls, is another manifestation resulting from vascular injury. In this setting, secondary segmental glomerulosclerosis is commonly observed.

The characteristic tubular lesion of CNI is cytoplasmic isometric vacuolization (Fig. 4.15). This lesion is typically focal and characterized by tubular epithelial cell cytoplasm that is densely packed with uniform, small vacuoles filled with PAS-negative material, a pattern more often seen in tacrolimus-associated toxicity. This represents a nonspecific finding because similar findings may be encountered in patients that have not been exposed to CNIs, particularly those receiving parenteral hyperosmolar agents, intravenous immunoglobulin (IVIG), or radiological contrast agents. Other tubular lesions associated with CNI toxicity include giant mitochondria (approximately half the size of the nucleus) and dystrophic calcifications. Owing to the lack of specificity, the diagnostic value of these other tubular findings is more limited.

There are no specific interstitial changes for CNI toxicity. Traditionally, CNI toxicity can result in so-called "striped fibrosis"; however, this finding lacks specificity because it can result from a variety of etiologies associated with ischemic injury (Fig. 4.16).

CNI toxicity can have several vascular manifestations, particularly in the arterioles (so-called "CNI arteriolopathy"). Acute toxicity can induce swelling and vacuolization of medial smooth muscle cells (Fig. 4.17). However, this is a nonspecific finding and may be seen in patients who have not received CNIs. Severe ischemic injury can also result in these morphological changes to medial smooth muscle cells; care must be taken to examine areas without tubular injury

for this feature. This swelling can progress to necrosis of the medial smooth muscle cells and subsequent replacement by hyalinized material. These events result in a characteristic feature of late CNI toxicity—arteriolar intramural hyaline depositions. These deposits can have a nodular morphology and stain strongly for PAS (Fig. 4.18). Afferent arterioles are thought to be primarily affected. Arteriolar hyalinosis is scored by the Banff system on a range from ah0 to ah3 and is based on the number of arterioles with focal or circumferential hyaline (Table 4.9). Severe CNI toxicity can also result in a TMA pattern of vascular injury, indistinguishable from other causes of TMA. Occasionally, hyperplasia of the juxtaglomerular apparatus may also be seen (Fig. 4.18a).

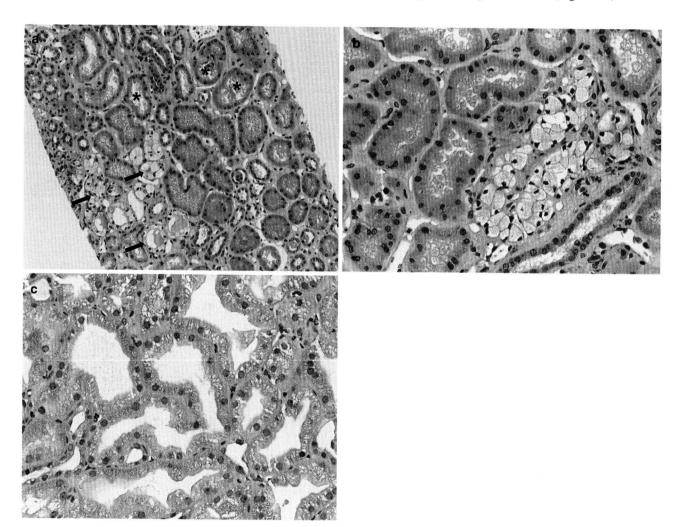

Fig. 4.15 (a) The epithelial cells in a few tubules (*arrows*) have clear vacuoles of similar size (isometric) in the cytoplasm, which impart a "foamy" appearance. Adjacent tubules show less specific features of ATN including apical blebbing. (b) On high magnification, the cytoplasm of some epithelial cells contains numerous clear small vacuoles of uniform size, characteristic of isometric vacuolization. This finding is commonly seen as a result of acute CNI toxicity, but is not pathognomonic because it can be seen in osmotic nephropathy, albeit it is usually more widespread in the latter. (c) Occasionally, nonspecific ATN can cause extensive vacuolization of the cytoplasm, mimicking isometric vacuolization. However, the vacuoles in these cases are more coarse and irregular and, therefore, should not be labeled as isometric vacuolization

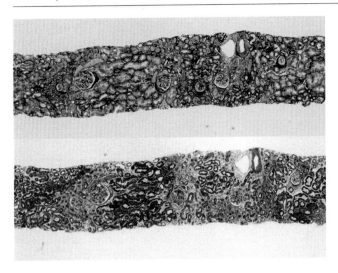

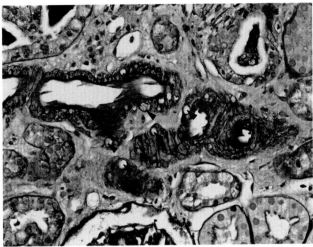

Fig. 4.16 Low-power view of the renal cortex shows alternating areas of tubulointerstitial fibrosis and nonscarred parenchyma, imparting a "striped" pattern. This is best appreciated in JMS- (*top*) and trichrome (*bottom*)-stained sections

Fig. 4.17 Cytoplasmic vacuolization or clearing of arterial smooth muscle cells (*arrowheads*) is a nonspecific finding often seen in severe cases of ischemic injury of any cause (PAS)

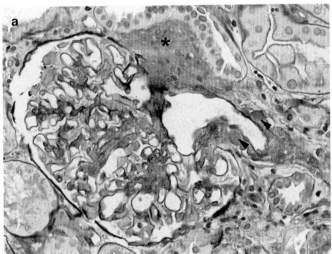

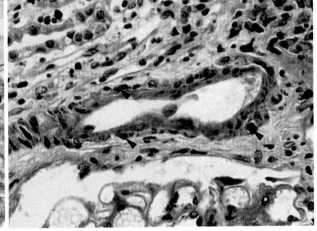

Fig. 4.18 (**a**) Necrotic smooth muscle cells are replaced by accumulations of PAS-positive hyaline material (*arrowheads*), which appear as nodules in the media of affected arterioles. The glomerulus shows hyperplasia of the juxtaglomerular apparatus (*asterisk*). Both findings have been attributed to chronic CNI toxicity (PAS stain). (**b**) On the trichrome stain, hyaline arteriolar deposits appear as bright red nodules (*arrowheads*)

Table 4.9 Scoring of arteriolar hyalinosis [3]

Banff score	Number of arterioles with hyalinosis
ah0	0
ah1	1 focal
ah2	>1 focal
ah3	At least 1 circumferential

4.8 Drug-Induced Acute Interstitial Nephritis

4.8.1 Morphological Features

The histological features of drug-induced acute interstitial nephritis (AIN) are essentially indistinguishable from type I ACR and, in many cases, definitive distinction between ACR and AIN is not possible. Morphological clues suggestive of a diagnosis of drug-induced AIN include inflammation centered in the outer medulla/corticomedullary junction with cortical sparing, and the presence of small and poorly formed non-necrotizing interstitial granulomas. Marked eosinophilia should raise suspicion for drug-induced AIN (Fig. 4.19) but is not a definitive diagnostic feature because ACR (especially with vascular rejection) may have pronounced eosinophilic infiltrates; furthermore, some cases of drug-induced AIN lack significant eosinophilia.

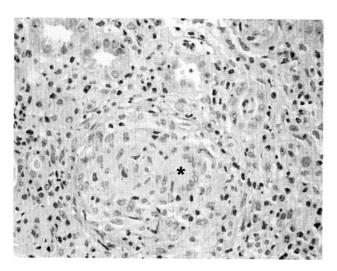

Fig. 4.19 Although increased interstitial eosinophils may be seen in ACR, especially severe ACR, brisk eosinophilic infiltrates as shown here are not a common feature of rejection and should raise suspicion for a drug-induced hypersensitivity reaction. In this example, the infiltrates are associated with a granuloma containing a multinucleated giant cell (*asterisk*)

4.9 Other Drugs

4.9.1 Rapamycin Toxicity

Rapamycin (sirolimus, everolimus, Rapamune) is an mTOR (mammalian target of rapamycin)–inhibitor immunosuppressive agent in use since the 1990s to allow lower doses of CNI and steroid and lessen the risk of chronic allograft nephropathy [21]. Although it is less nephrotoxic than CNIs, rapamycin nephrotoxicity does occur. Three different morphologies of rapamycin nephrotoxicity have been observed including focal segmental glomerulosclerosis, thrombotic microangiopathy, and rapamycin cast nephropathy.

4.9.2 Antiviral Drugs

Viral infections such as BK nephropathy are relatively common in renal transplant recipients. Antiviral agents such as cidofovir and leflunomide are concentrated in the proximal tubule and may result in acute tubular injury. In addition, these agents can precipitate into crystal resulting in crystal nephropathy. Other toxicities that can be observed include tubular mitochondriopathy (mega-mitochondria) and TMA.

4.10 Allograft Infections

4.10.1 Polyomavirus Virus Nephropathy

4.10.1.1 Clinical

The incidence of PVN in allograft kidneys is approximately 5 % and may present days to years post transplantation, but the most common timeframe for infection is between 2 months and 2 years post transplant [22]. The infection is generally limited to the kidney allograft and results from reactivation of latent polyomavirus (BK virus usually, rarely JC) present in the donor kidney in the setting of transplant immunosuppression. Clinical signs are nonspecific and can include allograft dysfunction with increased serum creatinine. Hematuria, proteinuria, and constitutional signs of infections such as fever and leukocytosis are usually absent. Because of the disease is limited to the kidney, diagnosis requires a renal biopsy.

4.10.1.2 Microscopic Features

The two common histological features of PVN are (1) epithelial intranuclear viral inclusions and (2) viral injury and lysis of tubular epithelial cells (Fig. 4.20). No cytoplasmic inclusions are present in PVN. Four discrete types and numerous hybrid variants of viral nuclear change can coexist in a single biopsy specimen. Focal involvement of tubules and collecting ducts by PVN is characteristic; occasionally, only distal nephron/medulla involvement is observed. Early disease stages may show no histological changes and may be detectable only by IHC. Two cores, including medulla, should be considered minimally adequate diagnostic material in the absence of definite pathological findings. Varying degrees of tubular injury may be present consisting of lysis and denudation of tubular epithelial cells. Tubular basement membranes are typically left intact. Parietal epithelial cells of Bowman capsule are occasionally affected and can be associated with the formation of pseudocrescents. Podocyte involvement is vanishingly rare.

Interstitial inflammation and fibrosis is variable and may range from none to abundant. When present, interstitial inflammation is mixed and includes lymphocytes, macrophages, and plasma cells. Prominent tubulitis can be present and may make distinction from ACR difficult (Fig. 4.21). Plasma cells may be prominent, including plasma cell tubulitis. Useful but unusual findings are intratubular granulomas, which are rare in rejection and should generate consideration for PVN. IF studies may show granular IgG or C4d staining on tubular basement membranes [23]. The proposed grading system of PVN is three tiered and based on the degree of polyomavirus replication and interstitial fibrosis (Table 4.10) [24].

PVN can be confirmed using IHC detection of the SV40 T antigen. Positive nuclear staining indicates viral replication (not virions themselves). A strong signal can be seen in cells without viral inclusions and absent in adjacent cells with viral inclusions. A single renal epithelial cell with positive nuclear staining (intensity $\geq$ 2+ out of 4) is sufficient for the diagnosis. By EM, polyomaviruses are found primarily in the nucleus. The virions are 30–45 nm and occasionally form crystalloid structures (Fig. 4.22).

In contrast to PVN, other viral infections are only very rarely encountered on renal transplant biopsies.

CMV infection is a systemic and symptomatic infection usually occurring 1–3 months after transplant [25]. CMV infection presents with fever, leukopenia, multiorgan dysfunction, and viremia. The gastrointestinal tract and lungs are most commonly affected. Kidney involvement is rare (5 %). Histological detection of CMV infection in the kidney is very rare and usually found in very focal tubular epithelial cells and occasionally endothelial cells and podocytes. Typical CMV nuclear and cytoplasmic inclusions are seen and can be associated with nodular- to granulomatous-appearing lymphoplasmacytic cell infiltrate. Diagnosis can be confirmed via IHC. Enveloped virions of 150 nm in diameter are observed under EM.

Rarely, adenovirus infection can occur in the allograft kidney [26]. The major histological features of adenovirus nephropathy are (1) viral inclusions in tubular epithelial cell nuclei, (2) severe tubular destruction including rupture of basement membranes and focal necrosis with neutrophils, (3) a plasmahistiocytic infiltrate with occasional granuloma formation, and (4) red cell casts in tubular lumens and focal interstitial hemorrhage (Fig. 4.23). The diagnosis can be confirmed with IHC studies. Nuclear and cytoplasmic virions approximately 75–80 nm in diameter can be observed via EM.

Other Infectious Etiologies Because of their immunosuppressed states, kidney transplant recipients are at an increased risk for infection with opportunistic organisms including bacteria (pyelonephritis) and systemic mycoses.

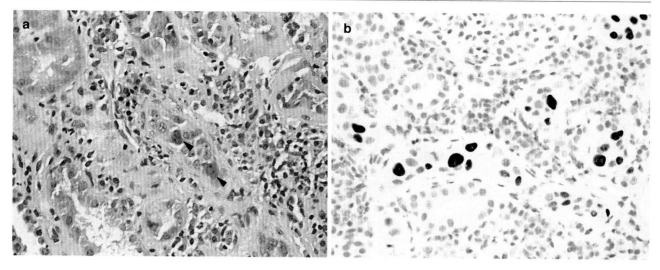

Fig. 4.20 (a) The nuclei of several epithelial cells are markedly enlarged and have a "ground-glass" appearance due to the presence of viral inclusions (*arrowheads*), which cause peripheral displacement of the nucleoli. There is an interstitial inflammatory cell infiltrate in the background that includes numerous plasma cells, and multiple foci of tubulitis (*arrows*). (b) SV40 immunostain on the same case shows strong nuclear positivity of the infected tubular epithelial cells, confirming the diagnosis of PVN

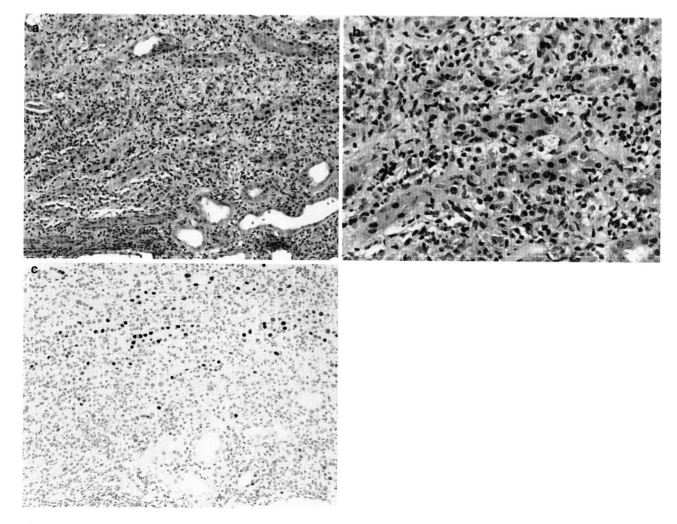

Fig. 4.21 (a) PVN is typically a focal or multifocal process; however, in severe cases, the involvement can be more diffuse. (b) On higher magnification, frequent foci of severe tubulitis often resulting in overrun of tubules are evident. Although nuclear epithelial atypia is present, no obvious viral inclusions are identified histologically and, therefore, a diagnosis of severe ACR needs to be considered. Because of the treatment implications, a low threshold for work-up of cases for PVN is recommended, particularly in patients with unknown BK status. (c) An SV40 immunostain confirms the diagnosis of PVN. It is important to remember that PVN and ACR can occur simultaneously, but such a combined diagnosis can be reliably established only in the presence of concurrent arteritis

Table 4.10 PVN grading criteria [24]

Stage	Viral replication	Tubules	Interstitial fibrosis (%)
A (early)	Viral replication (intranuclear inclusion bodies and/or positive SV40)	No viral acute tubular injury	<50
B (florid changes)	Marked viral replication (intranuclear inclusion bodies and/or positive SV40)	Virally induced acute tubular injury in one or more tubular cross sections	<50
C (late sclerosing changes)	Variable viral replication and tubule injury		>50

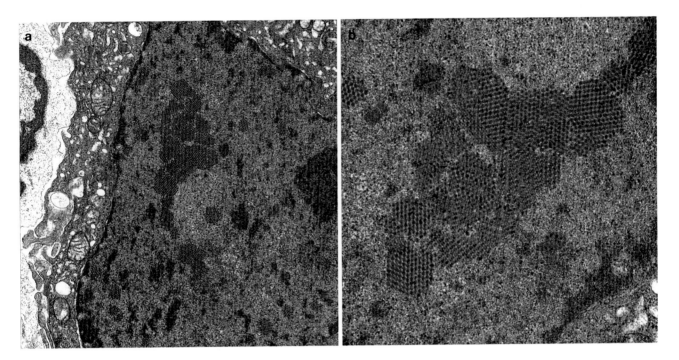

Fig. 4.22 (**a**) Ultrastructural appearance of an infected tubular epithelial cell with intranuclear virions. (**b**) Higher magnification allows better visualization of the intranuclear virions in regular parallel arrays

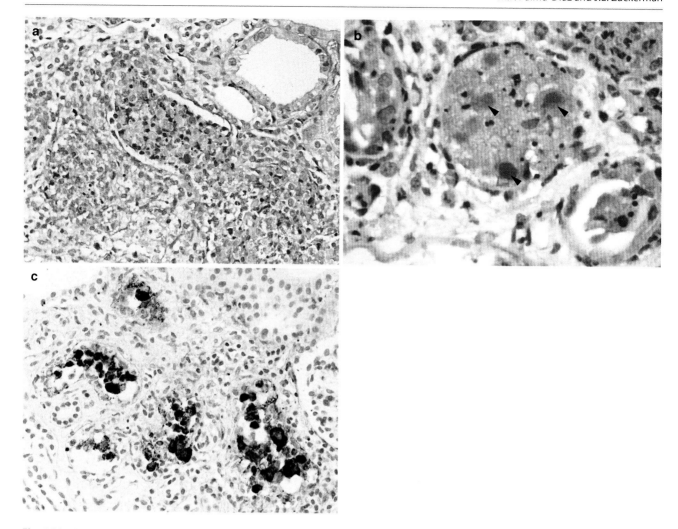

Fig. 4.23 (a) Adenovirus nephropathy causes prominent injury to the tubular lining, resulting in cellular necrosis and disruption of the basement membrane, often associated with vague granulomatous inflammation (PAS stain). (b) Adenoviral inclusions are basophilic and impart a smudgy appearance to the cell nuclei (*arrowheads*) (Courtesy of Dr. Ian Roberts, John Radcliffe Hospital, Oxford). (c) Immunostain for adenovirus showing predominantly nuclear but also cytoplasmic staining is confirmatory

4.11 Post-transplant Lymphoproliferative Disorder

PTLD is a lymphoid proliferation or lymphoma that develops secondary to immunosuppression in solid organ or bone marrow allograft recipients [27]. PTLD is a spectrum disorder ranging from early, Epstein-Barr virus (EBV)-driven polyclonal lymphoid proliferation to EBV-positive or -negative lymphomas of predominantly B-cell (85 %) and occasionally T-cell type (Table 4.11). PTLD is less common in kidney transplants than other solid organs with an incidence rate of approximately 1 %. See Chap. 9 for more information.

Table 4.11 WHO histological categories and subtypes of PTLD [26]

PTLD category	Histological subtype	Frequency (%)
Early lesions	Plasma cell hyperplasia	<5
	Infectious mononucleosis like	
Polymorphic PTLD		10–20
Monomorphic PTLD	B-cell PTLD	>60
	T-cell PTLD	<5
Classic Hodgkin		<5

WHO World Health Organization

4.11.1 Distinguishing PTLD from ACR

EBV detection is often a helpful ancillary study to distinguish PTLD from ACR. Of note, a small fraction (<10 %) of cells in ACR may be EBV positive. PTLD should be favored only when a large fraction of the infiltrating lymphocytes are positive for EBV. Other features that are suggestive of PTLD over ACR include "crowding out" of tubules by lymphoid infiltrate; lymphoid infiltrate extending beyond renal capsule; a uniform, large cell lymphoid infiltrate; mixed infiltrate with atypical large transformed lymphocytes and immunoblasts; necrosis of lymphocytes in the infiltrate; and a predominantly B-cell infiltrate.

4.12   Patterns of Chronic Change

Chronic changes in the allograft kidney result from a composite of interrelated processes including direct effects of chronic rejection, secondary effects of chronic rejection (decreased renal mass, ischemia, hypertension), chronic toxic/drug or ischemic injury, infections, recurrent/de novo glomerular disease, and systemic processes (hypertension, diabetes). There are relatively few specific chronic features of any of these entities; however, certain characteristic patterns of chronic changes are associated with various etiologies.

4.13   Chronic Antibody-Mediated Rejection

4.13.1 Clinical Features

Approximately 60 % of late allograft failure results from CAMR. CAMR has an insidious presentation with an average time for graft dysfunction of 7.3 years post transplant. Clinically, CAMR may be associated with stable graft function, indolent dysfunction, or acute dysfunction, manifesting as proteinuria greater than 0.5 g/dL.

4.13.2 Microscopic Features

Diffuse GBM duplication/multilayering known as *transplant glomerulopathy* (TG) (Fig. 4.24) is the pattern of glomerular injury most widely accepted as the chief manifestation of CAMR, and is more commonly seen in association with class II HLA antibodies. The GBM changes, best appreciated on PAS or JMS stains, may be segmental or global with or without mesangial cell interposition. Mesangial hypercellularity and matrix accumulation is generally mild. Segmental sclerosis may be present owing to chronic antibody-mediated glomerular injury or as a secondary phenomenon. Marked glomerular hypertrophy can also be observed. The glomerulitis of AAMR may also be observed concurrently. Importantly, no bona fide immune deposits should be present on IF or EM studies.

The most severely affected, nonsclerotic, glomerulus is used by the Banff classification to score TG [14]. The scoring is based on whether GBM changes can be visualized by LM or only at the ultrastructural level (Table 4.12).

TG of CAMR has similar morphological features to and, needs to be distinguished from, chronic TMA of any etiology, but particularly CNI toxicity. Additional features of CNI toxicity and clinical history are useful for distinguishing these other entities. Regardless of the cause, TG presents clinically with some degree of proteinuria.

Another characteristic finding of CAMR is multilamination of PTC basement membranes, which can be evaluated only on ultrastructural examination. However, this feature is not entirely specific for CAMR. The most specific criteria for PTC basement membrane lamination due to chronic AMR includes assessment of the 3 most severely affected of at least 15 PTCs via EM. These 3 should have at least five layers of lamination and 1 of the 3 should have at least seven (Fig. 4.25) (Table 4.13). The positive predictive value of this finding for CAMR is high when present in conjunction with other morphological features of CAMR.

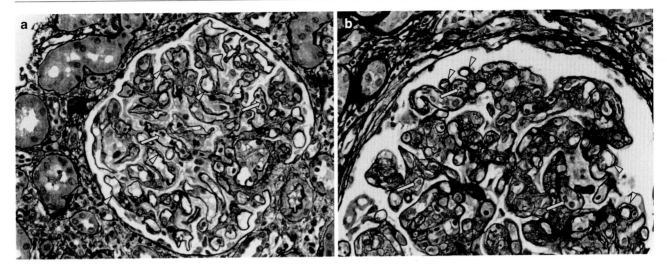

Fig. 4.24 (**a**, **b**) Glomeruli with widespread duplication of basement membranes or "double contours" of the capillary loops (*arrowheads*) are characteristic of chronic TG. This finding is best appreciated with silver stains and is often accompanied by variable increase in circulating leukocytes (*arrows*). These findings are indistinguishable from chronic thrombotic microangiopathy (JMS)

Table 4.12 Scoring of TG [16]

Banff Score		
cg0	No GBM double contours by LM or EM	
cg1	a	No GBM double contours by LM but GBM double contours (incomplete or circumferential) in at least three glomerular capillaries by EM with associated endothelial swelling and/or subendothelial electron-lucent widening
	b	One or more glomerular capillaries with GBM double contours in 1 nonsclerotic glomerulus by LM; EM confirmation is recommended if EM is available

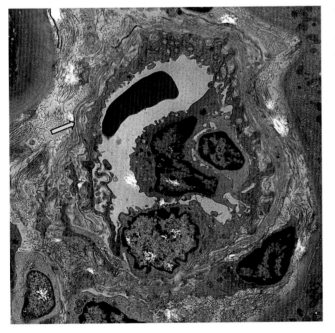

Table 4.13 Criteria for assessing CAMR ptc multilamination by EM [16]

At least 3 ptc with >5 layers of lamination
At least 1 ptc with >7 layers of lamination
15 ptc evaluated by EM

Fig. 4.25 A PTC shows multilayering of the basement membrane, a relatively specific finding of CAMR if there are at least seven layers of lamination in one PTC (*arrow*). The endothelium appears swollen and there are increased circulating leukocytes

4.13.3 Immunofluorescence

C4d staining of PTC in conjunction with the aforementioned morphological findings strongly suggests CAMR; however, lack of this finding should not dissuade the pathologist from such a diagnosis because a high proportion of patients with CAMR have no C4d at the time of biopsy (see Sect. 4.13.5). In this latter group, the process may be inactive [14].

Glomeruli with TG may show nonspecific staining for various immune reactants including IgM, C3, and fibrinogen. Strong granular staining for immunoglobulin or complement components should raise the possibility of an immune complex–mediated process. In this instance, ultrastructural confirmation is extremely helpful.

4.13.4 Electron Microscopy

EM plays a major role in the diagnosis of CAMR, given its higher sensitivity for detecting TG compared with LM, because it can disclose early changes including endothelial cell swelling, subendothelial widening due to accumulation of electron lucent material, and early neomembrane formation (Fig. 4.26). In addition, it allows visualization of multilayering of PTC basement membranes. Moreover, in cases with equivocal immune deposits on IF studies, it plays an important confirmatory role.

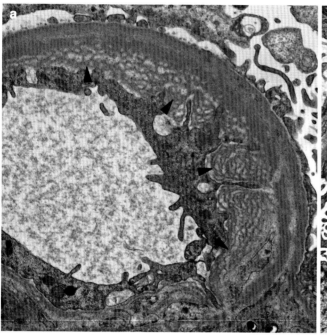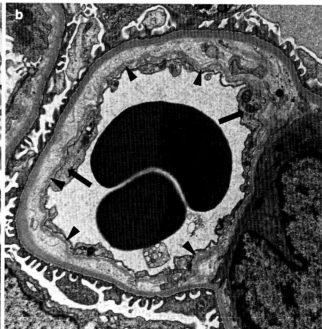

Fig. 4.26 (**a**) Ultrastructural appearance of TG, characterized by thickening of the subendothelial space due to accumulation of electron-lucent material and neomembrane formation (basement membrane multilayering) (*arrowheads*). (**b**) In early TG, the basement membrane changes (*arrowheads*) are more subtle and apparent only at the ultrastructural level. Often, these findings are accompanied by endothelial cell swelling with loss of fenestrations (*arrow*)

4.13.5 Diagnostic Criteria for CAMR

Similar to AAMR, the diagnosis of CAMR requires (1) histological evidence of chronic tissue injury, (2) evidence of current or recent antibody interaction with vascular endothelium, and (3) serological evidence of circulating antibodies to donor endothelium antigens (DSAs) (Table 4.14). If only two criteria are met (e.g., negative C4d or no DSA assay) the findings are interpreted as suspicious for CAMR. In the absence of evidence of current or recent antibody interaction with the endothelium, the term active should be omitted; in these cases, evidence of DSAs may be present at the time of the biopsy or at any prior time post transplantation.

Table 4.14 Banff criteria for chronic AAMR [16]

1. Histological evidence of chronic tissue injury (at least one or more)	TG (cg > 0), if no evidence of chronic thrombotic microangiopathy
	Severe PTC basement membrane multilayering (requires EM)
	Arterial intimal fibrosis of new onset, excluding other causes
2. Evidence of current or recent antibody interaction with vascular endothelium (at least one or more)	ptc C4d staining (C4d2, C4d3 on IF or C4d > 0 on IHC)
	At least moderate microvascular inflammation (g + ptc ≥ 2)
	Increased expression of ENDATs or other gene expression markers of endothelial injury in biopsy tissue
3. Serological evidence of DSAs	HLA, ABO, or other antigens

4.14 Patterns of Chronic Arteriolar Change

The major patterns of chronic arteriolar change are (1) arteriolar hyalinosis, (2) arteriolar intimal thickening without elastosis, and (3) arteriolar nephrosclerosis. These patterns are best appreciated on elastic-stained sections where the elastic lamina can be evaluated.

4.14.1 Arterial Intimal Fibrosis

Arterial intimal fibrosis can result from a variety of etiologies including chronic ACR, CAMR, and hypertension. The classic pattern of intimal fibrosis known as chronic active sclerosing transplant arteriopathy is thought to be primarily a result of "smoldering" cell-mediated rejection (Fig. 4.27). The arteriopathy results from accumulation of types I and III collagen in the subintimal space without elastosis. Rare to marked intimal mononuclear inflammation may be present as well as intimal myofibroblasts and foam cells. The overlying endothelial cells may appear "reactive" with underlying neomedia formation. Chronic rejection is favored in the absence of internal elastic lamina duplication. There are no specific features that can differentiate between chronic ACR and CAMR. The Banff classification score for arterial intimal fibrosis is based on the degree of luminal occlusion of the most involved artery (Table 4.15).

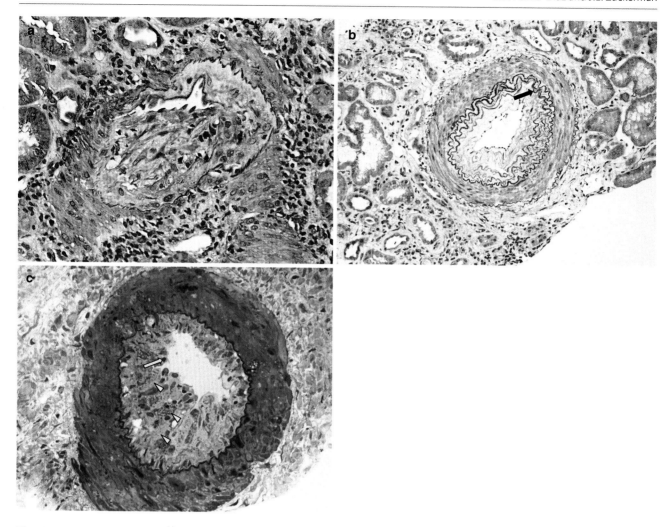

Fig. 4.27 (**a**) Expansion of the intima of this interlobular artery is shown by increases in cellularity and matrix. The cells in the intima consist of mononuclear inflammatory cells and mesenchymal cells. On this trichrome-elastic stain, there is no significant duplication of the internal elastic lamina, a finding that helps distinguish chronic transplant arteriopathy from arteriosclerosis secondary to hypertension (Trichrome-EVG stain). (**b**) Hypertension-induced changes in an artery result in thickening of the intima due to matrix deposition. In contrast to chronic allograft arteriopathy, there is duplication of the internal elastic lamina (*arrow*) and no associated inflammatory cell infiltration (Trichrome-EVG stain). (**c**) On this toluidine blue stain, there is intimal thickening predominantly due to increased cellularity. The cells in this example are primarily foam cells (*arrowheads*), but scattered mononuclear inflammatory cells are also seen (*arrow*). There is only mild matrix deposition (Toluidine stain)

Table 4.15 Scoring of arterial intimal fibrosis [3]

Banff score	Maximal % luminal narrowing of most affected artery
cv0	0
cv1	25
cv2	26–50
cv3	>50

4.14.2 Arteriolar Hyalinosis

In this pattern of chronic arteriolar change, amorphous, glassy and eosinophilic material is observed in the walls of renal arterioles resulting in thickened arteriolar walls and luminal narrowing. The major diagnostic considerations of this pattern of chronic change include chronic CNI toxicity, diabetes, and hypertension. This feature is scored as described earlier in Sect. 4.7.1.2 on CNI toxicity (ah scoring).

The location and morphology of the hyalinosis can provide clues to the underlying etiology. Arteriolar hyalinosis is an extremely common sequela of hypertension and diabetes and is usually primarily subendothelial and surrounded by an atrophic medial layer (Fig. 4.28). Occasionally, medial and transmural hyaline deposition can be observed. Primarily medial, peripheral, and adventitial nodular hyalinosis are more characteristic, although not pathognomonic of CNI toxicity. Combination changes are also common because many kidney transplant patients treated with CNIs also suffer from hypertension and/or diabetes.

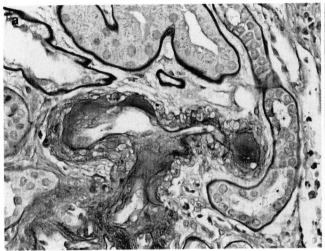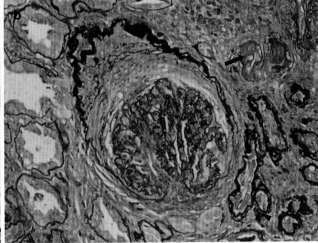

Fig. 4.28 (**a**) Arteriolar hyalinosis with primary subendothelial involvement (as opposed to medial) is a common nonspecific finding that may result from aging, hypertension, and/or diabetes mellitus (PAS; 400×). (**b**) In cases with severe arteriolar hyalinosis (*arrow*), there is marked narrowing of the lumen—often associated with TA (*arrowheads*) and interstitial fibrosis—and ischemic glomerular changes characterized by irregular wrinkling of the capillary walls and thickening of Bowman capsule as in this glomerulus (PAS stain, 200×)

4.14.3 Arteriolar Nephrosclerosis: Hypertension, Diabetes

The distinguishing morphological feature of arteriolar nephrosclerosis is concentric duplication of the arterial internal elastic lamina (fibroelastosis). There should be no, or only very few, inflammatory cells present. These features are not included in the Banff scoring system. The primary differential diagnosis for this lesion is chronic transplant arteriopathy; however, no duplication of the arterial internal elastic lamina should be observed in this setting.

4.15 Common, Nonspecific, Pathological Changes in the Allograft Kidney and Diagnostic Pitfalls

4.15.1 Subcapsular Fibrosis

The capsule of the native kidney contains penetrating vessels that supply the outer rim of the renal cortex. Circulation to these vessels is lost when a kidney is transplanted, resulting in atrophy and fibrosis of the subcapsular renal parenchyma in nearly all kidney allografts (Fig. 4.29). Inflammation and interstitial fibrosis in the subcapsular region should be excluded in the evaluation of the allograft kidney biopsy.

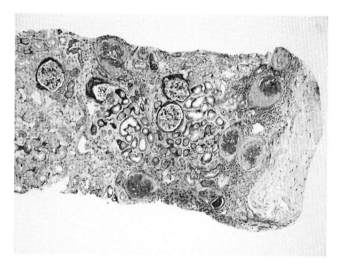

Fig. 4.29 Subcapsular scarring and inflammation is common and results from disruption of the capsular collateral circulation of the allograft following transplantation. This finding is nonspecific. Unawareness of this nonspecific finding may lead to overinterpretation of chronic changes in the biopsy or a misdiagnosis of rejection (PAS stain)

4.15.2 Inflammation in Areas of TA and Interstitial Fibrosis

Areas of TA and interstitial fibrosis of any etiology are often associated with mild to moderate chronic inflammatory cell infiltration (Fig. 4.5d). This inflammation is nonspecific and should not be considered evidence for rejection or infection (although it is included in the Banff "ti" score; see Sect. 4.3.1).

4.15.3 Inflammation Centered in the Corticomedullary Junction and Around Vessels

Inflammation can occasionally be observed prominently involving the corticomedullary junction (Fig. 4.30) or surrounding vessels. These patterns of inflammation are nonspecific and should not be overinterpreted as evidence for rejection or infection when present in isolation.

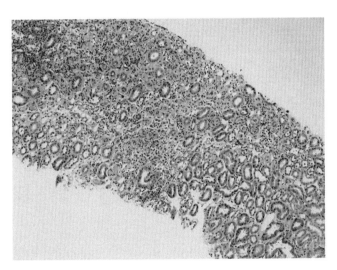

Fig. 4.30 Inflammation confined to the corticomedullary junction is a nonspecific finding and should not be interpreted as ACR or infection if there are no other associated features

4.15.4 Medulla

Medullary regions are of limited diagnostic value in the allograft biopsy. Inflammation here is nonspecific. Situations in which the medulla contains diagnostic material include (1) acute pyelonephritis, (2) C4d staining of medullary PTCs in AMR, and (3) polyomavirus infection; the medulla may occasionally have the only diagnostic material.

4.16 Recurrent Disease

The frequency of disease recurrence is difficult to ascertain accurately; however, in one study, recurrent glomerular disease was found to be the third most common cause of late graft failure [27]. Recurrence usually occurs within 12 months of transplantation, with some entities manifesting as early as 1 week. Symptomatic recurrences typically manifest with an increase in serum creatinine, proteinuria, and/or hematuria, but a significant proportion is subclinical. Virtually all forms of glomerulonephritis have been shown to recur in the allograft. The rates vary greatly, depending on the disease (Table 4.16) [29–31]. Biopsy determination of the primary cause of renal disease may be a necessary prerequisite for the accurate diagnosis of recurrent disease.

Table 4.16 Select recurrent diseases in the renal allograft [28–30]

Disease	Recurrence rate (%)	Diagnostic comments
Focal segmental glomerulosclerosis, primary type (idiopathic)	20–50	Early recurrence, particularly in children Diffuse foot process effacement (earliest manifestation) and podocyte detachment precede development of histological lesions by months
IgA nephropathy	9–61	Marked histological variability
Membranous nephropathy	7–44	Findings can be seen within 1 week post transplantation
Diabetic nephropathy	40	Diabetic changes may occur significantly earlier compared with native kidneys
Atypical hemolytic-uremic syndrome	20–90	Recurrence rate depends on underlying genetic abnormality
Dense deposit disease	90–100	Despite recurrence may have normal renal function and no/minimal proteinuria

References

1. John R, Herzenberg AM. Our approach to a renal transplant biopsy. J Clin Pathol. 2010;63:26–37.

2. Williams WW, Taheri D, Tolkoff-Rubin N, Colvin RB. Clinical role of the renal transplant biopsy. Nat Rev Nephrol. 2012;8:110–21.

3. Racusen LC, Solez K, Colvin RB, Bonsib SM, Castro MC, Cavallo T, et al. The Banff 97 working classification of renal allograft pathology. Kidney Int. 1999;55:713–23.

4. Schwarz A, Gwinner W, Hiss M, Radermacher J, Mengel M, Haller H. Safety and adequacy of renal transplant protocol biopsies. Am J Transplant. 2005;5:1992–6.

5. Solez K, Axelsen RA, Benediktsson H, Burdick JF, Cohen AH, Colvin RB, et al. International standardization of criteria for the histologic diagnosis of renal allograft rejection: the Banff working classification of kidney transplant pathology. Kidney Int. 1993;44: 411–22.

6. Solez K, Colvin RB, Racusen LC, Haas M, Sis B, Mengel M, et al. Banff 07 classification of renal allograft pathology: updates and future directions. Am J Transplant. 2008;8:753–60.

7. Nankivell BJ, Alexander SI. Rejection of the kidney allograft. N Engl J Med. 2011;364:485–6.

8. Mannon RB, Matas AJ, Grande J, Leduc R, Connett J, Kasiske B, et al. Inflammation in areas of tubular atrophy in kidney allograft biopsies: a potent predictor of allograft failure. Am J Transplant. 2010;10:2066–73.

9. Mengel M, Reeve J, Bunnag S, Einecke G, Jhangri GS, Sis B, et al. Scoring total inflammation is superior to the current Banff inflammation score in predicting outcome and the degree of molecular disturbance in renal allografts. Am J Transplant. 2009; 9:1859–67.

10. Tuazon TV, Schneeberger EE, Bhan AK, McCluskey RT, Cosimi AB, Schooley RT, et al. Mononuclear cells in acute allograft glomerulopathy. Am J Pathol. 1987;129:119–32.

11. De Freitas DG, Sellarés J, Mengel M, Chang J, Hidalgo LG, Famulski KS, et al. The nature of biopsies with "borderline rejection" and prospects for eliminating this category. Am J Transplant. 2012;12:191–201.

12. Marfo K, Lu A, Ling M, Akalin E. Desensitization protocols and their outcome. Clin J Am Soc Nephrol. 2011;6:922–36.

13. Lorenz M, Regele H, Schillinger M, Exner M, Rasoul-Rockenschaub S, Wahrmann M, et al. Risk factors for capillary C4d deposition in kidney allografts: evaluation of a large study cohort. Transplantation. 2004;78:447–52.

14. Mauiyyedi S, Crespo M, Collins AB, Schneeberger EE, Pascual MA, Saidman SL, et al. Acute humoral rejection in kidney transplantation: II. Morphology, immunopathology, and pathologic classification. J Am Soc Nephrol. 2002;13:779–87.

15. Regele H, Exner M, Watschinger B, Wenter C, Wahrmann M, Osterreicher C, et al. Endothelial C4d deposition is associated with inferior kidney allograft outcome independently of cellular rejection. Nephrol Dial Transplant. 2001;16:2058–66.

16. Haas M, Sis B, Racusen LC, Solez K, Glotz D, Colvin RB, et al. Banff 2013 meeting report: inclusion of C4d-negative antibody-mediated rejection and antibody-associated arterial lesions. Am J Transplant. 2014;14:272–83.

17. Haas M, Rahman MH, Racusen LC, Kraus ES, Bagnasco SM, Segev DL, et al. C4d and C3d staining in biopsies of ABO- and HLA-incompatible renal allografts: correlation with Histologic findings. Am J Transplant. 2006;6:1829–40.

18. Bravou V, Galliford J, McLean A, Willicombe M, Taube D, Cook HT, et al. A case of chronic antibody-mediated rejection in the making. Clin Nephrol. 2013;80:306–9.

19. El-Zoghby ZM, Stegall MD, Lager DJ, Kremers WK, Amer H, Gloor JM, et al. Identifying specific causes of kidney allograft loss. Am J Transplant. 2009;9:527–35.

20. Naesens M, Kuypers DRJ, Sarwal M. Calcineurin inhibitor nephrotoxicity. Clin J Am Soc Nephrol. 2009;4:481–508.

21. Stallone G, Infante B, Schena A, Battaglia M, Ditonno P, Loverre A, et al. Rapamycin for treatment of chronic allograft nephropathy in renal transplant patients. J Am Soc Nephrol. 2005;16:3755–62.

22. Babel N, Volk H-D, Reinke P. BK polyomavirus infection and nephropathy: the virus-immune system interplay. Nat Rev Nephrol. 2011;7:399–406.

23. Bracamonte E, Leca N, Smith KD, Nicosia RF, Nickeleit V, Kendrick E, et al. Tubular basement membrane immune deposits in association with BK polyomavirus nephropathy. Am J Transplant. 2007;7:1552–60.

24. Sar A, Worawichawong S, Benediktsson H, Zhang J, Yilmaz S, Trpkov K. Interobserver agreement for Polyomavirus nephropathy grading in renal allografts using the working proposal from the 10th Banff Conference on Allograft Pathology. Hum Pathol. 2011;42:2018–24.

25. De Keyzer K, Van Laecke S, Peeters P, Vanholder R. Human cytomegalovirus and kidney transplantation: a clinician's update. Am J Kidney Dis. 2011;58:118–26.

26. Florescu MC, Miles CD, Florescu DF. What do we know about adenovirus in renal transplantation? Nephrol Dial Transplant. 2013;28:2003–10.

27. Swerdlow SH, Campo E, Harris NL, Jaffe ES, Pileri S, Stein H. WHO classification of tumours of haematopoietic and lymphoid tissues. Lyon: IARC Press; 2008. p. 343.

28. Cruzado JM. Recurrent glomerulonephritis and risk of renal allograft loss. N Engl J Med. 2002;347:1531–2; author reply 1531–2.

29. Kidney Disease: Improving Global Outcomes (KDIGO) Working Group. KDIGO clinical practice guideline for the care of kidney transplant recipients. Am J Transplant. 2009;9 Suppl 3:S1–155.

30. Sprangers B, Kuypers DRK. Recurrence of glomerulonephritis after renal transplantation. Transplant Rev (Orlando). 2013;27:126–34.

31. Menn-Josephy H, Beck Jr LH. Recurrent glomerular disease after kidney transplantation. Front Biosci (Elite Ed). 2015;7:135–48.

Liver Transplant Pathology

Bita V. Naini and Samuel W. French

Histopathologic evaluation plays an integral role in the overall assessment of the liver transplant. Pathologists are often asked to evaluate donor liver biopsies to assist in the determination of whether a marginal donor liver is suitable for transplantation. In addition, histopathologic assessment of allograft liver biopsies plays an important role in identifying the cause of allograft dysfunction and therefore in initiation of the appropriate therapeutic intervention. A detailed histopathologic evaluation is mandated, including histologic comparison with any previous biopsies as well as incorporation of all pertinent clinical, laboratory, and imaging findings with histologic assessment.

B.V. Naini, MD (✉)
Department of Pathology and Laboratory Medicine, David Geffen School of Medicine at the University of California, Los Angeles, 10833 Le Conte Avenue, 27-061C7 CHS, Los Angeles, CA, 90095-1732, USA
e-mail: bnaini@mednet.ucla.edu

S.W. French, MD, PhD
Department of Pathology and Laboratory Medicine, David Geffen School of Medicine at the University of California, Los Angeles, 10833 Le Conte Avenue, 13-145 CHS, Los Angeles, CA, 90095-1732, USA

© Springer International Publishing Switzerland 2016
W.D. Wallace, B.V. Naini (eds.), *Practical Atlas of Transplant Pathology*, DOI 10.1007/978-3-319-23054-2_5

5.1 Evaluation of Donor Biopsies

Donor biopsies are often evaluated to determine the extent of steatosis. There are two different forms of steatosis—macrovesicular and microvesicular—with the macrovesicular form divided into large droplet and small droplet. Large droplet macrovesicular steatosis is generally defined as one large fat vacuole that occupies more than half of the cell and displaces the nucleus to the cell periphery (Fig. 5.1). In comparison, small droplet macrovesicular steatosis is defined as fat vacuoles that are smaller than half of the cell and do not displace the nucleus (Fig. 5.2). The term microvesicular steatosis is used when innumerable tiny lipid vesicles are diffusely distributed throughout the cytoplasm, giving it a foamy appearance [1–3]. The extent of steatosis is estimated as the percentage of liver parenchyma that is replaced by steatosis (Fig. 5.3). It is typically the extent of large droplet macrovesicular steatosis that is clinically significant because more or less than 30 % of this type of steatosis has been shown to be an independent risk factor for reduced short-term graft survival. The exact amount of steatosis that precludes an organ for transplantation is rather center-dependent and depends on various donor and recipient factors. Small droplet macrovesicular steatosis and microvesicular steatosis do not predictably result in graft dysfunction, and in many centers such as ours they are not used to determine graft usage. In our practice, we estimate the amount of fat in routine hematoxylin and eosin (H&E) staining (either requested as frozen section or rush permanent evaluation), and we do not perform any special fat stains. It is important that the biopsy specimen is freshly obtained and that frozen sections are evaluated immediately or the biopsy is placed in formalin for fixation, since exposure to air or saline can significantly alter the morphology and hamper the evaluation of the biopsy.

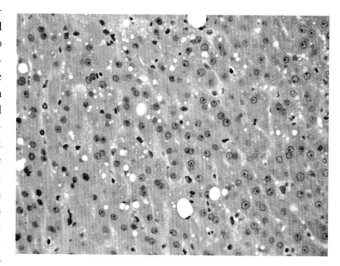

Fig. 5.2 Small droplet macrovesicular steatosis is shown as small fat droplets that occupy less than half of the cytoplasm and do not displace the nucleus. The presence of this type of steatosis in a donor organ generally does not preclude that organ from being used for transplantation. A few large droplet macrovesicular vesicular steatosis is also seen here

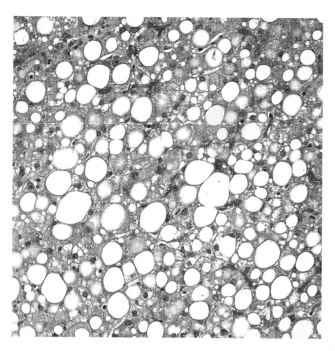

Fig. 5.1 Large droplet macrovesicular steatosis is shown as fat droplets occupying greater than half of the cytoplasm and displacing the nucleus

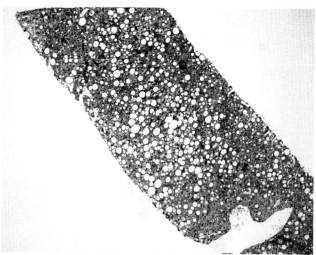

Fig. 5.3 Donor biopsy. This potential donor liver biopsy shows extensive large droplet macrovesicular steatosis (>30 % of parenchyma). This amount of large droplet macrovesicular steatosis in a potential donor liver would generally make this liver unsuitable for transplantation

5.2 Allograft Rejection

Acute cellular rejection (ACR) is the most common type of rejection and the most common complication in the early post-transplant period. The diagnosis is based on three main histopathologic features: (1) mixed but predominantly mononuclear portal inflammation containing activated lymphocytes, neutrophils, and eosinophils; (2) subendothelial inflammation of portal and/or central veins (i.e., endotheliitis); and (3) bile duct inflammation and damage (Figs. 5.4, 5.5, and 5.6). The minimum diagnostic criteria for ACR are generally accepted as the presence of at least two of these features [4]. However, because these findings may vary considerably in different areas of the graft, it is recommended that a minimum of five portal tracts and at least two sections at different levels be examined when evaluating allograft biopsies [5].

Once the diagnosis of acute rejection has been established based on the above criteria, the Banff schema (Table 5.1) is applied to grade the severity of acute rejection [6]. The schema assesses the severity of inflammation, combined with morphologic evidence of rejection-related ischemia, which is the final mechanism of allograft failure in ACR. A descriptive grading of rejection is rendered based on an overall evaluation of the parameters listed in Table 5.1.

In general, mild and moderate acute rejections are distinguished based on the extent of the portal inflammation, whereas the presence of perivenular inflammation and associated hepatocellular necrosis is used to distinguish severe acute rejection from the lower grades (Fig. 5.7). In most mild cases of ACR, the inflammatory infiltrate is limited to the portal tracts. The presence of prominent interface hepatitis indicates either a more severe form of ACR, a late form of ACR (see later description), or another concomitant cause of hepatitis. If more than one inflammatory condition is affecting the allograft (e.g., acute rejection and viral hepatitis), it is extremely difficult if not impossible to determine the relative contribution of each injury to the severity of the changes.

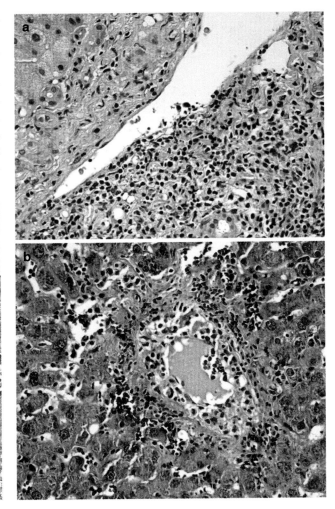

Fig. 5.5 (**a, b**) Acute cellular rejection. Endotheliitis. The prominent subendothelial lymphocytic infiltrate is lifting up and detaching the overlying endothelium from the basement membrane. Endotheliitis most commonly involves portal veins (**a**) but can also be seen in central veins (**b**). Endotheliitis is considered the most specific diagnostic feature of acute cellular rejection (Image **b** Courtesy of Charles Lassman, MD, PhD)

Fig. 5.4 Acute cellular rejection. The portal inflammatory infiltrate is mixed and consists predominantly of lymphocytes, including large activated immunoblasts with large nuclei, prominent nucleoli, and abundant eosinophilic cytoplasm. Other inflammatory cells include eosinophils, plasma cells, macrophages, and occasional neutrophils. This portal infiltrate may range from mild to severe and can involve a few to all sampled portal tracts

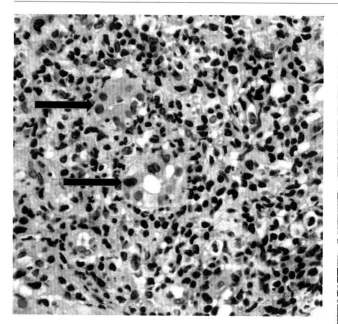

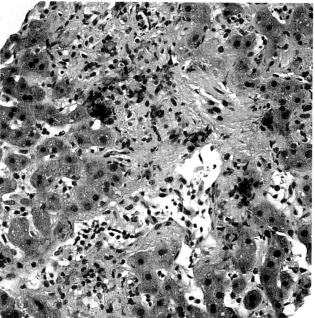

Fig. 5.6 Acute cellular rejection. Bile duct injury (*arrows*) is shown as lymphocytic infiltration of the duct epithelium accompanied by epithelial cell injury with nuclear enlargement, overlapping nuclei, loss of nuclear polarity, cytoplasmic vacuolization, and luminal disruption

Fig. 5.7 Acute cellular rejection. The presence of perivenular inflammation and associated hepatocellular necrosis in this case would make this a severe case of acute cellular rejection. Central vein endotheliitis is also present; however, its presence is not necessary for a diagnosis of severe acute cellular rejection

Table 5.1 Banff schema for grading liver allograft acute rejection

Global assessment	Criteria
Indeterminate	Portal inflammatory infiltrate that fails to meet the criteria for the diagnosis of acute rejection
Mild	Rejection infiltrate in a minority of the triads that is generally mild and confined to the portal spaces
Moderate	Rejection infiltrate, expanding most or all the triads
Severe	As above for moderate, with spillover into periportal areas and moderate to severe perivenular inflammation that extends into the hepatic parenchyma and is associated with perivenular hepatocyte necrosis

5.2.1 Late Acute Rejection

This form of rejection refers to a type of cellular rejection that occurs several months after transplantation and may show different histologic features as compared with typical ACR described earlier. Alternative names include centrizonal/parenchymal rejection, hepatitic variant of rejection, or atypical rejection. It is characterized by a hepatitic pattern of liver injury and can mimic hepatitis closely [7, 8]. Perivenular inflammation (central perivenulitis) is commonly seen, which may or may not be associated with centrilobular hepatocyte injury and necrosis (Fig. 5.8). Late acute rejection is considered a diagnosis of exclusion, and complete serologic studies (including rare forms of viral hepatitis such as hepatitis E) must be performed to rule out other etiologies of hepatitis. Of note, hepatitis E is an uncommon but increasingly recognized cause of acute and chronic hepatitis in the developed countries and should be considered in any post–liver transplant patient with a hepatitic pattern of injury. In general however, if central perivenulitis is present in less than 50 % of the lobules, the diagnosis of late acute rejection is favored [9].

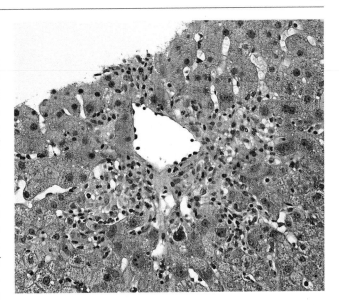

Fig. 5.8 Central perivenulitis is characterized by an inflammatory infiltrate surrounding the central vein, which may or may not be associated with centrilobular hepatocyte injury, dropout, and necrosis. In the presence of characteristic portal changes of rejection, central perivenulitis is a sign of severe acute cellular rejection, whereas isolated central perivenulitis is a histologic finding that may be seen in late acute rejection

5.2.2 Plasma Cell Hepatitis (PCH)

PCH is an immune-mediated post-transplant histologic pattern of injury. It is characterized by the presence of plasma cell–rich portal and lobular inflammatory infiltrates, including central perivenulitis, which closely resembles autoimmune hepatitis in the native liver (Fig. 5.9) [10]. While the pathophysiology is somewhat unclear, PCH is generally considered a form of rejection and is a negative prognostic factor for graft and patient outcomes. Patients with this pattern of injury are more likely to be resistant to increased immunosuppression and have an increased risk of fibrosis and graft loss [11–13].

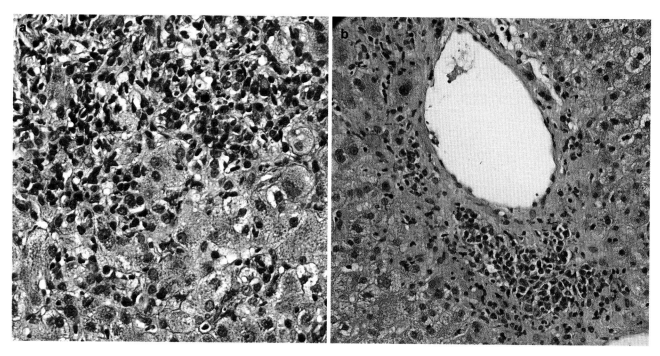

Fig. 5.9 (**a, b**) Plasma cell hepatitis. Numerous plasma cells are seen among the portal and periportal inflammatory infiltrate (**a**) as well as in pericentral areas (**b**) of this post-transplant liver biopsy. This pattern of injury is generally considered a form of rejection and imparts a negative prognostic factor for graft function and patient outcome

5.2.3 Chronic Rejection (CR)

In comparison to other solid organ transplants (such as heart, lung, and kidney) in which CR may affect 30–50 % of allograft recipients, CR affects only 3–5 % of liver transplant recipients. Although late CR is considered an irreversible, progressive disease that leads to graft loss, early CR is considered potentially reversible [14]. Early CR is identified by degenerative changes of the biliary epithelium, even before duct loss. These include uneven spacing of biliary epithelial cells, loss of nuclear polarity, and increased cytoplasmic eosinophilia (Fig. 5.10). Late CR is characterized by bile duct loss involving greater than 50 % of portal tracts (Fig. 5.11). Other lobular features that may be seen in later phases of CR include clusters of pigmented foamy macrophages, canalicular cholestasis, pericentral hepatocyte atrophy, and/or ballooning and perivenular fibrosis (Figs. 5.12, 5.13, and 5.14). While foam cell obliterative arteriopathy is the characteristic feature of CR, this finding is only rarely seen in needle core biopsies (Fig. 5.15). The minimum diagnostic criteria for histopathologic diagnosis of CR are defined as follows [15]: (1) the presence of bile duct atrophy/senescence affecting most of the bile ducts, with or without bile duct loss (early CR), (2) foam cell obliterative arteriopathy (OA) with accumulation of foamy, lipid-laden histiocytes within the myointimal layer, or (3) loss of interlobular bile ducts in at least 50 % of the portal tracts (late CR).

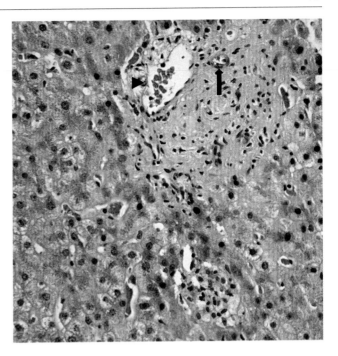

Fig. 5.11 Chronic rejection. This biopsy showed loss of bile ducts in the majority of portal tracts. The portal tract here shows a branch of hepatic artery (*arrow*) and portal vein (*arrowhead*) but no interlobular bile duct. Immunostain for cytokeratin 7 or 19 may be used to help confirm the bile duct loss

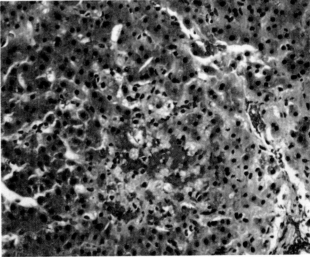

Fig. 5.12 Chronic rejection. Cluster of pigmented macrophages within the lobule with cholestasis may be seen in chronic rejection

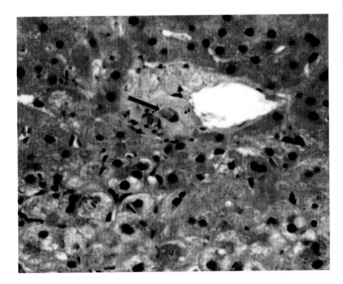

Fig. 5.10 Early chronic rejection with bile duct atrophy/senescence (*arrow*) characterized by uneven epithelial spacing, loss of nuclear polarity, nuclear atypia, and increased cytoplasmic eosinophilia. Note that there is no ductular reaction or portal infiltrate (*Courtesy of* Charles R. Lassman, MD, PhD)

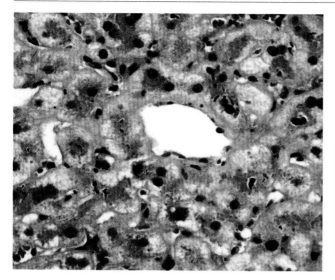

Fig. 5.13 Chronic rejection. Pericentral cholestasis is seen with canalicular bile plugging and cholate stasis with feathery degeneration

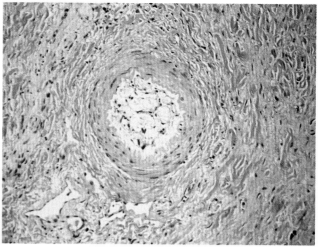

Fig. 5.15 Chronic rejection. Foam cell obliterative arteriopathy is the hallmark feature of chronic rejection and is characterized by intimal thickening with accumulation of lipid-laden foamy macrophages that can cause luminal narrowing and obstruction. This lesion is rarely seen in biopsy material

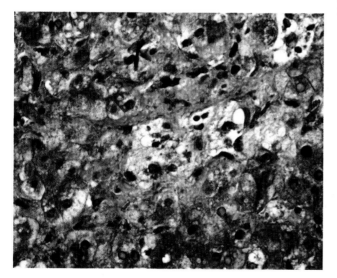

Fig. 5.14 Late chronic rejection. Trichrome stain highlights perivenular fibrosis in this case of late chronic rejection

5.2.4 Antibody-Mediated Rejection (AMR)

AMR is becoming increasingly recognized in liver allografts. However, it remains a controversial area because its diagnostic criteria and histologic features have not been fully established. In general, AMR may be considered if other etiologies of allograft dysfunction have been excluded and if donor-specific antibodies (DSAs) are discovered in the patient's serum. Histologic features that have been reported include portal edema and neutrophilic inflammation with ductular reaction (i.e., features similar to those of bile duct obstruction), hepatocellular necrosis (i.e., features of ischemic injury) as well as portal vein endothelial cell hypertrophy, portal eosinophilia, and eosinophilic central venulitis (Fig. 5.16). Diffuse C4d deposition in the portal vein and sinusoids, demonstrated by immunohistochemistry and/or immunofluorescence, has been described in cases with clinical suspicion of AMR in the presence of DSAs (Fig. 5.17) [16–18]. However, the C4d stain remains a nonspecific stain, and its clinical utility remains unclear because positivity has also been reported in cases of ACR, CR, recurrent hepatitis B and C, biliary obstruction, vascular thrombosis, and even normal allograft livers [19]. The Banff schema consensus guidelines for diagnosis of AMR and C4d interpretation in liver allograft are expected to be released in the near future.

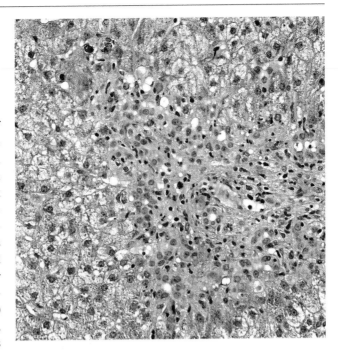

Fig. 5.16 Antibody-mediated rejection. The portal tract shows expansion by ductular reaction and edema, resembling features of bile duct obstruction. In this case, biliary obstruction was ruled out by imaging studies while the patient showed persistent signs of allograft dysfunction along with positive serum DSAs, and was determined to have AMR

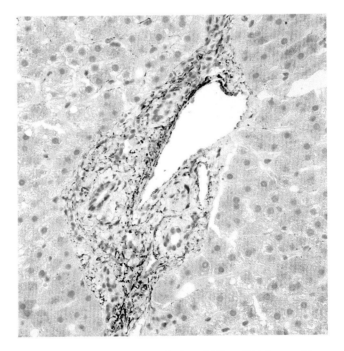

Fig. 5.17 Antibody-mediated rejection. Diffuse C4d immunohistochemical staining of greater than 50 % of portal veins/capillaries has been reported in cases with clinical suspicion of AMR in the presence of serum DSAs

5.3   Recurrent Disease

Recurrent disease is a major cause of graft dysfunction. Examples of some of the more common recurrent diseases follow.

5.3.1   Recurrent Hepatitis C

Recurrent hepatitis C is a major differential diagnosis of ACR, including late acute rejection. Early recurrence is characterized by a predominance of lobular activity with frequent apoptotic bodies (Figs. 5.18 and 5.19). Later there is a transition to predominantly portal infiltrates and interface hepatitis typical of chronic hepatitis C in native livers. The histologic feature that is very useful in determining whether acute rejection is present in the setting of recurrent hepatitis C is endotheliitis. However, it may not be present in late acute rejection. Table 5.2 contains histologic features helpful in differentiating ACR from recurrent hepatitis C.

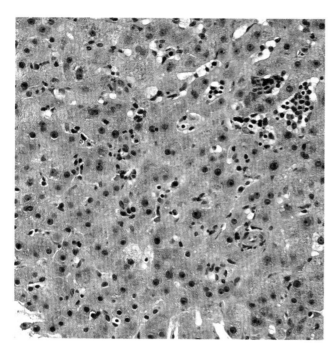

Fig. 5.18   Recurrent hepatitis C viral infection. Early recurrence manifests primarily as a lobular hepatitis with scattered clusters of lymphocytes

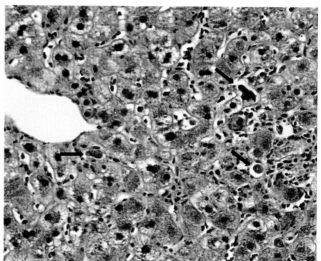

Fig. 5.19   Recurrent hepatitis C viral infection. Apoptotic hepatocytes (*arrows*) are a common feature of early recurrence

Table 5.2   Histologic features of acute rejection versus those of recurrent hepatitis C and primary biliary cirrhosis (PBC)

Histologic feature	Acute cellular rejection	Recurrent hepatitis C	Primary biliary cirrhosis
Portal inflammation	Mixed, with activated lymphocytes, plasma cells, neutrophils, and frequent eosinophils	Predominantly lymphocytic; may be nodular. Eosinophils are inconspicuous or few	Lymphoplasmacytic, sparse or dense; may be centered on bile duct
Bile ducts	Lymphocytic infiltration with epithelial injury. A very good indication of ACR, if it involves >50 % of portal tracts	Even if lymphocytic infiltration is present, it is mild and/or focal	Variable infiltration by lymphocytes and variable injury from mild to florid duct lesions
Portal vein endotheliitis	Present	Absent or mild and focal	Absent
Interface activity	Variable (often seen in moderate to severe ACR and in late ACR)	Minimal in early recurrence. Present in later phases	Ductular reaction and/or interface activity is often present
Lobular activity/injury	May be present in severe ACR but also in late ACR	Predominant in early recurrence, variable later	Variable; generally minimal
Apoptotic hepatocytes	Absent to occasional	Frequent	Absent to occasional
Central perivenulitis (with or without central vein endotheliitis)	May be present in severe ACR or late ACR	Absent or focal/mild, without endotheliitis	Generally uninvolved

5.3.2 Fibrosing Cholestatic Hepatitis (FCH)

This is a rare and aggressive form of viral hepatitis infection that occurs in patients with severe immunosuppression. It has been described in patients with both hepatitis B and C. Histologically, FCH is characterized by marked hepatocellular injury in the form of lobular disarray and ballooning changes in addition to prominent intracellular and canalicular cholestasis, ductular reaction, and periportal and pericellular/sinusoidal fibrosis (Fig. 5.20) [20–23]. There is generally a paucity of portal and lobular inflammatory infiltrate. This is a diagnosis of exclusion and requires clinicopathologic correlation with a markedly elevated viral load and exclusion of bile duct obstruction by imaging studies.

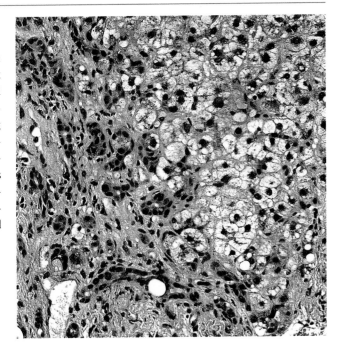

Fig. 5.20 Fibrosing cholestatic hepatitis (FCH). Irregular portal expansion with ductular reaction and diffuse parenchymal ballooning changes and cholestasis can be seen. Note the presence of ductular reaction and the relative paucity of inflammatory infiltrate. Histologically, FCH may mimic bile duct obstruction. However, the latter is not generally accompanied by extensive hepatocellular injury/ballooning and instead may show prominent portal edema

5.3.3   Primary Biliary Cirrhosis (PBC)

The histopathologic findings of recurrent PBC are identical to those seen in native livers. Given the presence of bile duct

injury and/or loss in cases of recurrent PBC (Fig. 5.21), the differential diagnosis between acute and chronic rejection can be challenging. (See Tables 5.1 and 5.2 for histologic features that are helpful in this distinction.)

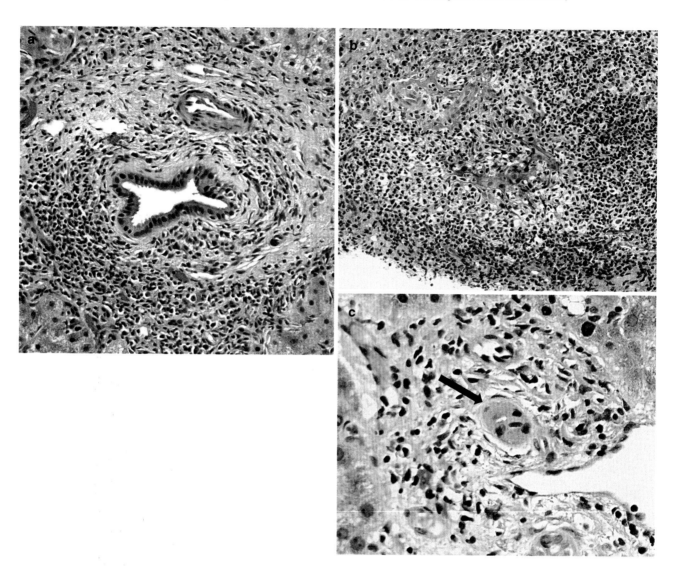

Fig. 5.21 (a–c) Recurrent primary biliary cirrhosis (PBC). Note the robust portal inflammatory infiltrate and florid duct lesions (a, b) in this case of recurrent PBC, 2 years post-transplant. Note the atrophic bile duct (*arrow*) with minimal inflammation in a different case of a late recurrent PBC (c). The distinction from acute and early chronic rejection can be difficult in such cases. See Tables 5.1 and 5.2 for some histologic clues (*Photo Courtesy of* Charles Lassman, MD, PhD)

5.3.4 Primary Sclerosing Cholangitis (PSC)

Recurrent PSC cannot be reliably distinguished from other forms of biliary obstruction on biopsy specimens, and cholangiography is essential in establishing a diagnosis. In addition, distinguishing PSC from chronic rejection can be challenging because both PSC and chronic rejection may result in atrophy and loss of interlobular bile ducts. However, features of PSC that are not typically seen in chronic rejection include portal inflammation, ductular reaction, and portal fibrosis (see Table 5.3).

Table 5.3 Histologic features of chronic rejection (CR) versus those of recurrent hepatitis C, primary biliary cirrhosis (PBC), and primary sclerosing cholangitis (PSC)

Histologic feature	Chronic rejection	Recurrent hepatitis C	Primary biliary cirrhosis	Primary sclerosing cholangitis
Portal inflammation	Minimal inflammation	Nodular lymphocytic infiltrate	Variable, from minimal to robust	Variable
Bile ducts	Early CR: atrophy and senescence Late CR: absent	Normal to mild lymphocytic infiltration	May be normal, atrophic, or absent; inflammatory lesions may be present	May be normal, atrophic, or absent; Periductal fibrosis or collagenous scars may be present
Portal fibrosis	None or minimal fibrous expansion	Variable, portal fibrosis progressing to bridging fibrosis and cirrhosis	Variable, portal fibrosis progressing to bridging fibrosis and cirrhosis	Variable, portal fibrosis progressing to bridging fibrosis and cirrhosis
Interface activity	None or minimal	Present	Variable	Variable
Ductular reaction	Absent	May be present	Generally present	Generally present
Lobular activity/ injury	Late CR: Kupffer cell aggregates, cholestasis, perivenular fibrosis may be seen in late CR	Variable: apoptotic cells are usually present; small lymphocytic aggregates may also be present	May be similar to CR with Kupffer cell aggregates and cholestasis	May be similar to CR with Kupffer cell aggregates and cholestasis

5.4 Infections

5.4.1 Cytomegalovirus Hepatitis (CMV)

CMV can infect hepatocytes, endothelial cells, and bile duct epithelial cells. Infected cells have an enlarged nucleus with an eosinophilic inclusion surrounded by a clear halo [24].

The cytoplasm often also contains eosinophilic granular inclusions. Adjacent liver sections may show clusters of neutrophils forming characteristic neutrophilic "microabscesses" (Figs. 5.22 and 5.23). In fact, this finding in isolation is considered a reasonable indication for performing immunohistochemical analysis to evaluate for CMV.

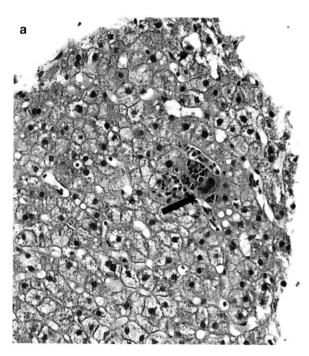
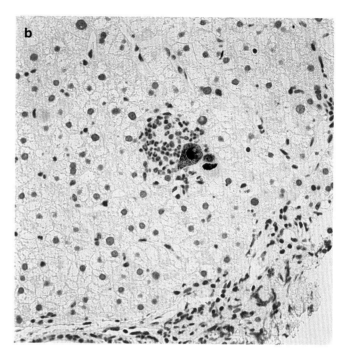

Fig. 5.22 (**a, b**) CMV infection. Note the infected cell with an eosinophilic nuclear inclusion (*arrow*) seen adjacent to a cluster of inflammatory neutrophils forming a characteristic neutrophilic "microabscess" (**a**). Immunohistochemistry highlights CMV- infected cells (**b**). Characteristic CMV inclusions might not be present on H&E stain, and therefore immunohistochemical staining for CMV should be considered in any allograft liver biopsy with a clinical and/or histologic suspicion for CMV infection

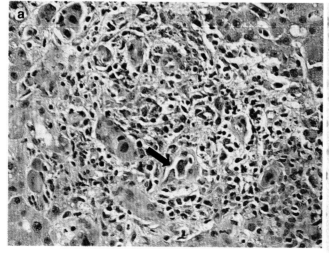
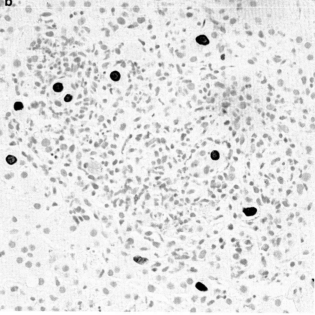

Fig. 5.23 (**a, b**) CMV infection. CMV may infect any many cell types including endothelial cells, bile duct epithelial cells, or hepatocytes. In this case, many CMV-infected cells are seen in this portal tract (**a**) and are highlighted by immunohistochemistry (**b**). Note the presence of both cytoplasmic and nuclear eosinophilic inclusions (*arrow* in **a**)

5.4.2   Adenovirus Hepatitis

Adenoviral infection is characterized by patchy nonzonal coagulative necrosis. Typically, hepatocytes peripheral to the necrosis demonstrate smudgy nuclei with chromatin margination (Fig. 5.24).

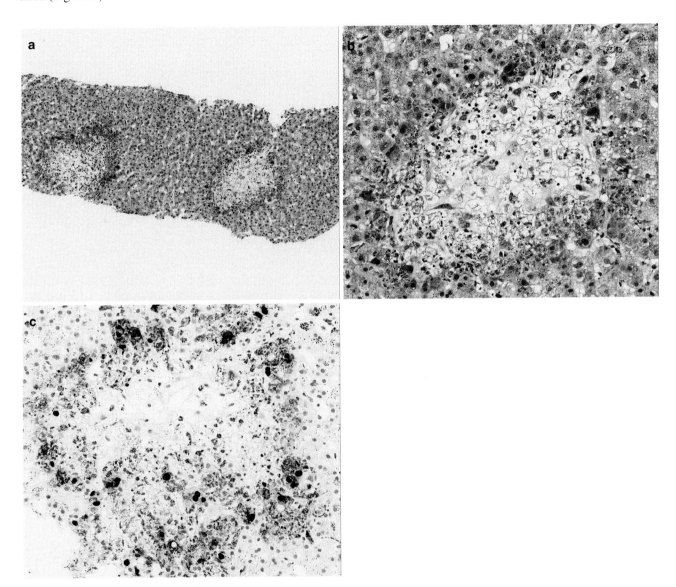

Fig. 5.24 (**a–c**) Adenovirus infection. This infected allograft liver shows patchy hepatocellular necrosis. Note that there is no zonal distribution for the areas of necrosis (**a**). The adenovirus-infected cells are seen at the edges of the necrotic area and show smudged nuclei and chromatin margination (**b**). Immunohistochemical analysis highlights the adenovirus inclusions within infected cells surrounding the necrotic area (**c**)

5.4.3 Herpes Simplex (HSV) and Varicella-Zoster (VZV) Hepatitis

HSV and VZV infections occur secondary to reactivation from latency any time post-transplant. These infections are similar histologically and show variable degrees of hepatocellular necrosis (up to massive) with the typical nuclear features of herpes infection, including multinucleation with molding of nuclei, margination of chromatin, and glassy nuclear inclusions (Fig. 5.25).

5.4.4 Epstein Bar Virus (EBV) Hepatitis

EBV infection is also seen as a reactivation from a previous infection. It might present as a range of histologic changes from mild EBV hepatitis seen as portal and sinusoidal lymphocytic infiltrate to post-transplant lymphoproliferative disorder (PTLD) (see later description). In situ hybridization testing for EBV-encoded RNA (EBER) is helpful.

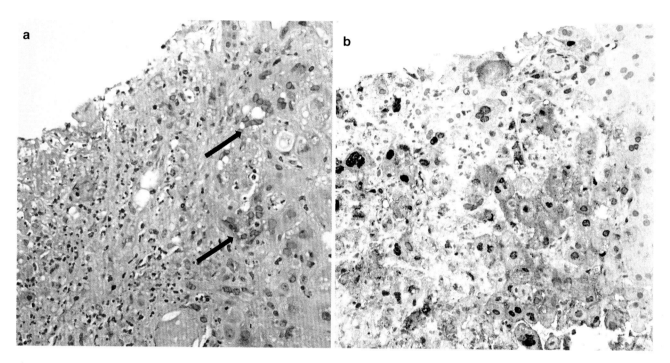

Fig. 5.25 (**a, b**) HSV infection. Infected hepatocytes (*arrows*) demonstrate multinucleation and nuclear chromatin margination. Focal necrosis is also present (**a**). Immunohistochemical study demonstrates numerous infected hepatocytes (**b**)

5.5   Other Complications

5.5.1   Preservation/Reperfusion Injury

This is one of the most common causes of allograft dysfunction within the first several weeks after transplantation. It is a general term that refers to the injury that may happen at any time, starting from the donor organ's acquisition, harvesting, and implantation into the recipient. It includes the cold ischemic time of the donor organ as well as injury related to postperfusion. Histologically, it is typically seen as pericentral sinusoidal congestion with neutrophilic infiltration of lobules accompanied by necrotic/apoptotic hepatocytes (Fig. 5.26).

5.5.2   Vascular Thrombosis

This is one of the most serious post-transplant technical complications and most often involves the hepatic artery. It most frequently occurs during the first several weeks post-transplant and less frequently 1–3 years after transplantation. Vascular compromise may be seen as pericentral hepatocellular damage, manifested as hepatocellular ballooning with cholate stasis and cholestasis (Fig. 5.27). In more severe cases, pericentral hepatocellular necrosis is present (Fig. 5.28). Other causes of pericentral necrosis in liver allografts include ischemic shock from hypovolemia or sepsis. Patients with sepsis or intra-abdominal infection have a characteristic pattern of injury, so-called subacute nonsuppurative cholangitis, also known as cholangitis lenta (Fig. 5.29) [25, 26].

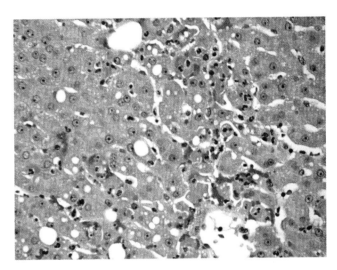

Fig. 5.26 Preservation/reperfusion injury is seen as sinusoidal congestion with neutrophilic inflammation and associated patchy hepatocyte necrosis/apoptosis

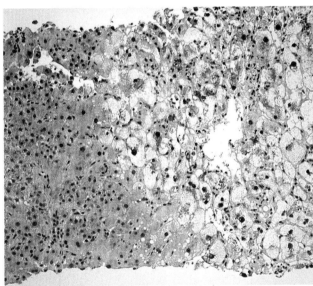

Fig. 5.27 Vascular thrombosis. Pericentral hepatocellular ballooning is seen in this patient with hepatic artery thrombosis

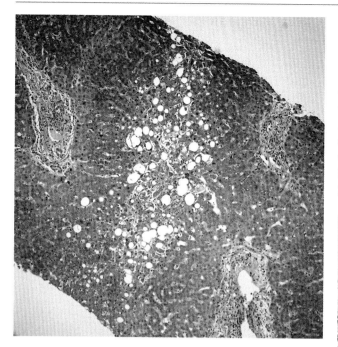

Fig. 5.28 Vascular thrombosis. This biopsy displays pericentral hepatocyte necrosis/apoptosis in a patient with hepatic artery thrombosis

5.5.3 Biliary Strictures/Bile Duct Obstruction

Biliary tract complications are a common source of dysfunction in the liver allograft. Histologic features include portal expansion with edema (neutrophilic), inflammatory infiltrate of portal tracts, and bile ductular reaction (Fig. 5.30). It is important to note that biopsies may show histologic features of mechanical obstruction when the initial imaging is negative for obstruction. Furthermore, bile duct obstruction can be a focal process, and therefore histologic features may not be seen in a biopsy from a nonaffected area.

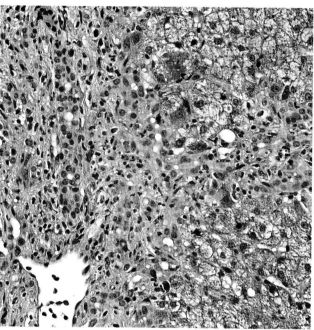

Fig. 5.30 Biliary stricture/bile duct obstruction. Features of bile duct obstruction (portal edema, ductular reaction, and neutrophilic infiltrates) are seen in this patient with a post-transplant biliary stricture

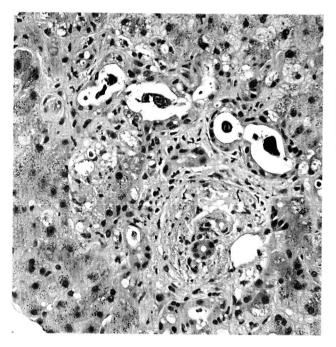

Fig. 5.29 Subacute nonsuppurative cholangitis (cholangitis lenta). This finding of dilated periportal ductules filled with inspissated bile has been generally associated with sepsis and/or intra-abdominal infection. Note that there is minimal portal inflammation and no portal edema

5.5.4 Adverse Drug Reaction

As in nontransplant patients, all forms of drug injury can be seen, including hepatitis and cholestasis. One type of change that is commonly seen in liver allograft is the presence of pseudo–ground-glass hepatocytes (Fig. 5.31) [27]. These deposits closely resemble the ground-glass inclusions of chronic hepatitis B infection. Immunostains for hepatitis B surface antigen may be helpful if there is any clinical concern and serologic testing is not available. Whether the drug injury alone accounts for the allograft dysfunction may not be clear.

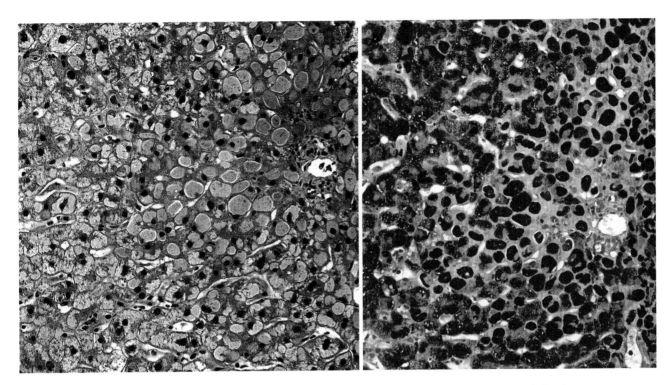

Fig. 5.31 (**a, b**) Pseudo–ground-glass hepatocytes. These hepatocytes show pale eosinophilic cytoplasmic inclusions that are displacing the nucleus to the side. This histologic feature may be seen in immunosuppressed patients on multiple medications and is commonly seen in allograft liver biopsies (**a**). Pseudo–ground-glass hepatocytes are associated with the accumulation of abnormal forms of glycogen, as demonstrated here by PAS stain (**b**)

5.5.5 Post-transplant Lymphoproliferative Disease (PTLD)

PTLD may present as an atypical portal and/or a lobular infiltration by mononuclear inflammatory cells, or a mass-forming lesion indistinguishable from lymphoma. It is commonly seen in the presence of EBV detected in tissue (Fig. 5.32). See Chap. 9 for more details.

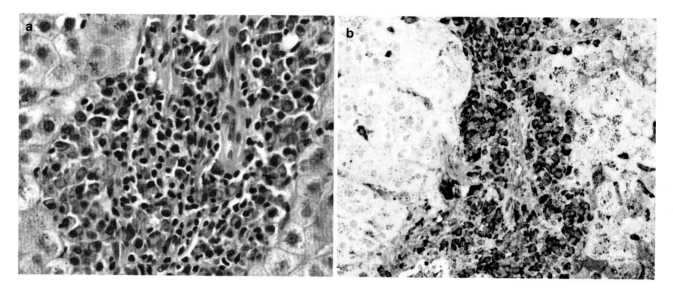

Fig. 5.32 (**a**, **b**) PTLD. Neoplastic plasmacytoid portal infiltrates are seen with little interface activity in this case of PTLD (**a**). The neoplastic cells in this case show light chain kappa restriction, as highlighted by immunohistochemistry (**b**)

References

1. Brunt EM. Surgical assessment of significant steatosis in donor livers: the beginning of the end for frozen-section analysis? Liver Transpl. 2013;19:360–1.
2. Brunt EM, Tiniakos DG. Histopathology of nonalcoholic fatty liver disease. World J Gastroenterol. 2010;16:5286–96.
3. Yersiz H, Lee C, Kaldas FM, Hong JC, Rana A, Schnickel GT, et al. Assessment of hepatic steatosis by transplant surgeon and expert pathologist: a prospective, double-blind evaluation of 201 donor livers. Liver Transpl. 2013;19:437–49.
4. International Working Party. Terminology for hepatic allograft rejection. Hepatology. 1995;22:648–54.
5. Liapis H, Wang HL. Pathology of solid organ transplantation. Heidelberg: Springer; 2011. p. xii.
6. Banff schema for grading liver allograft rejection: an international consensus document. Hepatology. 1997;25:658–63.
7. Akamatsu N, Sugawara Y, Tamura S, Keneko J, Matsui Y, Hasegawa K, et al. Late-onset acute rejection after living donor liver transplantation. World J Gastroenterol. 2006;12:6674–7.
8. Florman S, Schiano T, Kim L, Maman D, Levay A, Gondolesi G, et al. The incidence and significance of late acute cellular rejection (>1000 days) after liver transplantation. Clin Transplant. 2004;18:152–5.
9. Krasinskas AM, Demetris AJ, Poterucha JJ, Abraham SC, et al. The prevalence and natural history of untreated isolated central perivenulitis in adult allograft livers. Liver Transpl. 2008;14:625–32.
10. Khettry U, Huang WY, Simpson MA, Pomfret EA, Pomposelli JJ, Lewis WD, et al. Patterns of recurrent hepatitis C after liver transplantation in a recent cohort of patients. Hum Pathol. 2007;38:443–52.
11. Demetris AJ, Sebagh M. Plasma cell hepatitis in liver allografts: variant of rejection or autoimmune hepatitis? Liver Transpl. 2008;14:750–5.
12. Fiel MI, Agarwal K, Stanca C, Elhajj N, Kontorinis N, Thung SN, et al. Posttransplant plasma cell hepatitis (de novo autoimmune hepatitis) is a variant of rejection and may lead to a negative outcome in patients with hepatitis C virus. Liver Transpl. 2008;14:861–71.
13. Fiel MI, Schiano TD. Plasma cell hepatitis (de-novo autoimmune hepatitis) developing post liver transplantation. Curr Opin Organ Transplant. 2012;17:287–92.
14. Banff Working Group, Demetris AJ, Adeyi O, Bellamy CO, Clouston A, Charlotte F, Czaja A, et al. Liver biopsy interpretation for causes of late liver allograft dysfunction. Hepatology. 2006;44:489–501.
15. Demetris A, Adams D, Bellamy C, Blakolmer K, Clouston A, Dhillon AP, et al. Update of the International Banff Schema for Liver Allograft Rejection: working recommendations for the histopathologic staging and reporting of chronic rejection. An International Panel. Hepatology. 2000;31:792–9.
16. Haas M, Sis B, Racusen LC, Solez K, Glotz D, Colvin RB, Castro MC. Banff 2013 meeting report: inclusion of c4d-negative antibody-mediated rejection and antibody-associated arterial lesions. Am J Transplant. 2014;14:272–83.
17. Hubscher SG. Antibody-mediated rejection in the liver allograft. Curr Opin Organ Transplant. 2012;17:280–6.
18. O'Leary JG, Michelle Shiller S, Bellamy C, Nalesnik MA, Kaneku H, Jennings LW, et al. Acute liver allograft antibody-mediated rejection: an inter-institutional study of significant histopathological features. Liver Transpl. 2014;20:1244–5.
19. Taner T, Stegall MD, Heimbach JK. Antibody-mediated rejection in liver transplantation: current controversies and future directions. Liver Transpl. 2014;20:514–27.
20. Dixon LR, Crawford JM. Early histologic changes in fibrosing cholestatic hepatitis C. Liver Transpl. 2007;13:219–26.
21. Narang TK, Ahrens W, Russo MW. Post-liver transplant cholestatic hepatitis C: a systematic review of clinical and pathological findings and application of consensus criteria. Liver Transpl. 2010;16:228–35.
22. Satapathy SK, Sclair S, Fiel MI, Del Rio MJ, Schiano T. Clinical characterization of patients developing histologically-proven fibrosing cholestatic hepatitis C post-liver transplantation. Hepatol Res. 2011;41:328–39.
23. Xiao SY, Lu L, Wang HL. Fibrosing cholestatic hepatitis: clinico-pathologic spectrum, diagnosis and pathogenesis. Int J Clin Exp Pathol. 2008;1:396–402.
24. Lautenschlager I, Halme L, Höckerstedt K, Krogerus L, Taskinen E. Cytomegalovirus infection of the liver transplant: virological, histological, immunological, and clinical observations. Transpl Infect Dis. 2006;8:21–30.
25. Lefkowitch JH. Bile ductular cholestasis: an ominous histopathologic sign related to sepsis and "cholangitis lenta". Hum Pathol. 1982;13:19–24.
26. Lin CC, Sundaram SS, Hart J, Whitington PF. Subacute nonsuppurative cholangitis (cholangitis lenta) in pediatric liver transplant patients. J Pediatr Gastroenterol Nutr. 2007;45:228–33.
27. Wisell J, Boitnott J, Haas M, Anders RA, Hart J, Lewis JT, Abraham SC, Torbenson M. Glycogen pseudoground glass change in hepatocytes. Am J Surg Pathol. 2006;30:1085–90.

Small Bowel Transplant Pathology

6

Jamie Koo and Hanlin L. Wang

Small bowel transplantation (SBT) is increasingly used in the treatment of irreversible intestinal failure in both pediatric and adult patients. However, experience with SBT is relatively limited compared with that with other solid organ transplants, because early attempts in the 1960s and 1970s were primarily unsuccessful with most patients dying within days. It was not until the 1990s when advances in surgical techniques and immunosuppression regimens allowed for extended survival after transplantation [1]. Types of SBT include isolated small intestinal transplants (with or without colon), combined intestinal-liver transplants, multivisceral transplants (including small intestine with duodenum, liver, pancreas, and stomach), and modified multivisceral transplants (multivisceral transplants without liver and with or without stomach).

Because of the presence of commensal bacterial flora intrinsic to the small intestine, as well as the presence of abundant lymphoid tissue and innate and adaptive immune systems that are necessary to keep these microorganisms in check, the immunology of the small intestine is dynamic and complex. This poses great challenges for immunosuppression after transplantation. These unique complexities explain the high rates of rejection and infection seen after SBT and contribute greatly to long-term graft and patient survivals, which still remain low compared with that for other solid organ transplants. Based on data from 1998 to 2013, the 1- and 5-year graft survival rates were 78.6 and 48.0 % for isolated intestinal graft recipients and 70.6 and 48.9 % for combined intestinal-liver graft recipients, respectively [2]. Patient survival rates vary, with the lowest in adult intestinal-liver graft recipients (69.1 and 46.1 % for 1 and 5 years) and the highest in pediatric isolated intestinal graft recipients (89.2 and 81.4 % for 1 and 5 years).

The major barriers to long-term patient outcome are post-transplant complications, most notably acute cellular rejection (ACR), chronic rejection, infection, medication effects, and post-transplant lymphoproliferative disorder (PTLD). Histological evaluation of mucosal biopsies from transplanted bowel is essential in diagnosing these complications and, therefore, appropriate management of these patients. Usually, biopsies are obtained either as surveillance/protocol biopsies (in the absence of symptoms) or to evaluate the etiology of clinical symptoms such as fever, diarrhea, abdominal pain, and weight loss, among others. The diagnostic features of these major post-transplant complications are discussed in detail in this chapter.

J. Koo, MD • H.L. Wang, MD, PhD (✉)
Department of Pathology and Laboratory Medicine, David Geffen School of Medicine at the University of California, Los Angeles, Los Angeles, CA, USA
e-mail: hanlinwang@mednet.ucla.edu

© Springer International Publishing Switzerland 2016
W.D. Wallace, B.V. Naini (eds.), *Practical Atlas of Transplant Pathology*, DOI 10.1007/978-3-319-23054-2_6

6.1 Acute Cellular Rejection

ACR is a relatively common complication, with an incidence of 39 % in the first 12 months and 44 % by 24 months after transplantation [3]. In fact, it is the leading cause of graft failure in the first 2 months after transplantation. Clinical symptoms may include increased ostomy output, fever, nausea, vomiting, abdominal pain, and diarrhea. In general, the higher the grade of ACR, the longer the duration of the rejection episode. Endoscopic findings suggestive of ACR range from mucosal edema, erythema, friability, and focal ulcerations to a granular mucosal pattern with diffuse ulcerations, mucosal sloughing, and loss of peristalsis. ACR can be a focal finding and can affect the bowel in an unequal distribution in the proximal and distal segments. Thus, multiple biopsies should be obtained from both normal- and abnormal-appearing areas of the graft, as well as from native bowel, if possible [4]. Biopsies from mucosa adjacent to the stoma should be avoided, because nonspecific changes can be seen in this area.

6.1.1 General Histological Features of ACR and Grading System

The key histological features in the diagnosis of ACR in graft biopsies include:

1. Increased apoptotic activity in crypt epithelium.
    (a) Apoptotic bodies are characterized by fragmented/disintegrated and pyknotic nuclei, sometimes surrounded by a rim of clear cytoplasm, or clusters of nuclear dusts/debris within eosinophilic cytoplasm.
    (b) Small isolated fragments of nuclear chromatin should not be counted as apoptotic bodies.
    (c) Single, tiny, dotlike basophilic mucin granules in the cytoplasm of epithelial cells with well-pre-

served nuclei should not be counted as apoptotic bodies.
    (d) Ten consecutive, ideally well-oriented and longitudinally sectioned, crypts are counted. If the mucosa is cross-sectioned, all the linear cross sections between the mucosal surface and the muscularis mucosae should be counted as one crypt.
    (e) Epithelial apoptosis associated with ACR is typically observed at the base of crypts. Apoptotic activity occurring in surface lining cells should not be counted.
    (f) Normal grafts and native bowel typically show fewer than two apoptotic bodies per ten consecutive crypts.
2. Mixed lamina propria inflammatory cell infiltrates consisting predominantly of mononuclear cells with small and activated lymphocytes. Eosinophils and neutrophils can be prominent.
3. Epithelial injury ranging from reactive changes (such as loss of mucin, nuclear enlargement and hyperchromasia, increased mitotic figures, cytoplasmic basophilia, villous blunting, crypt architectural distortion, edema, and congestion), focal crypt withering, crypt loss/dropout, and erosion to ulceration.

ACR involvement is often patchy and histological findings on mucosal biopsies are often variable along the length of the graft. Thus, diagnostic features may sometimes be seen only in one biopsy in a set from multiple biopsy sites. The current grading schema into no ACR (grade 0), indeterminate for ACR (IND), mild ACR (grade 1), moderate ACR (grade 2), and severe ACR (grade 3) is based on criteria set forth by Wu et al. [5] and Ruiz et al. [6] and is summarized in Table 6.1. The histological features, differential diagnoses, and potential diagnostic pitfalls are further described in Tables 6.2, 6.3, 6.4, and 6.5 (Figs. 6.1, 6.2, 6.3, and 6.4). It should be mentioned that mild to severe arteritis may be present in the grafts in the setting of moderate and severe ACR, but this feature cannot be detected on mucosal biopsies.

Table 6.1 Histological grading of ACR in SBT biopsies

Grade of ACR	Apoptotic bodies per 10 consecutive crypts (n)	Epithelial injury	Lamina propria inflammation
No ACR	≤ 2	None	Normal components
Indeterminate	3–5	Minimal, usually focal	Minimal, usually localized
Mild	≥ 6	Mild, usually focal	Mild, usually localized
Moderate[a]	≥ 6 and confluent[b]	Focal crypt dropout, focal mucosal erosion	Moderate, usually extensive
Severe[a]	Variable in residual crypts	Extensive crypt dropout, extensive erosion and/or ulceration	Moderate to severe, extensive

[a]A varying degree of arteritis may be present in the setting of moderate and severe ACR, but this feature is not evident in superficial mucosal biopsies
[b]Confluent apoptosis involves all or the vast majority of the epithelial cells forming the crypt

Table 6.2 Indeterminate for ACR (Fig. 6.1)

Histological features
Increased crypt apoptotic activity: three to five apoptotic bodies per ten consecutive crypts
May show minimal epithelial injury, usually focal, characterized by reactive changes such as loss of mucin, nuclear enlargement and hyperchromasia, cytoplasmic basophilia, mild villous blunting, and others
Intact surface epithelium
May show a minimal increase in the number of lamina propria inflammatory cells, consisting predominantly of mononuclear cells. Activated lymphocytes may be present
Differential diagnosis
Mild ACR, which may show similar histological findings but with at least six apoptotic bodies per ten consecutive crypts
Infectious enteritis, which may show increased apoptotic activity but may also show more neutrophils and more severe epithelial injury disproportionate to apoptotic activity. Correlation with laboratory studies, such as serologies, stool studies, cultures, polymerase chain reaction, immunohistochemistry, and others, may be necessary
Medication effect (see Sect. 6.1.4)
Potential diagnostic pitfalls
Diagnosis of indeterminate for ACR implies that features of rejection are present but insufficient for diagnosis of mild rejection and, thus, should not be used in the context of nonspecific inflammation or infection
Intraepithelial lymphocytes, eosinophils, or neutrophils should not be mistaken for apoptotic bodies

Table 6.3 Mild ACR (Fig. 6.2)

Histological features
Increased crypt apoptotic activity: ≥ 6 apoptotic bodies per 10 consecutive crypts
May show mild epithelial injury, usually focal, characterized by reactive changes such as loss of mucin, nuclear enlargement and hyperchromasia, cytoplasmic basophilia, mild villous blunting, and others
Intact surface epithelium
May show a mild increase in the number of lamina propria inflammatory cells, consisting predominantly of mononuclear cells. Activated lymphocytes, eosinophils, and neutrophils may be present
Differential diagnosis
Indeterminate for ACR, which would have similar findings but with <6 apoptotic bodies per 10 consecutive crypts
Moderate ACR, which may show confluent apoptosis but would also show focal crypt dropout and/or focal erosion of the mucosa
Infectious enteritis (see Sect. 6.4)
Medication effect (see Sect. 6.1.4)
Potential diagnostic pitfalls
Biopsies from or near the stoma or anastomosis may show nonspecific inflammation, villous architectural change, and epithelial injury, which should not be used to evaluate for rejection
Intraepithelial lymphocytes, eosinophils, or neutrophils should not be mistaken for apoptotic bodies

Table 6.4 Moderate ACR (Fig. 6.3)

Histological features
Increased crypt apoptotic activity: more prominent than that seen for mild ACR in general. Apoptosis can be confluent to involve all or the vast majority of the epithelial cells in individual crypts
Focal crypt withering and/or dropout
Reactive and regenerative changes
Moderate increase in the number of lamina propria inflammatory cells, usually extensive, consisting predominantly of mononuclear cells. Activated lymphocytes, eosinophils and neutrophils are usually present. Neutrophilic cryptitis may be seen
May show focal mucosal erosion
Differential diagnosis
Severe ACR, which would show more extensive crypt dropout with more extensive erosion or ulceration
Infectious enteritis, especially cytomegalovirus (CMV) enteritis with ulceration
Medication effect (see Sect. 6.1.4)
Potential diagnostic pitfalls
Biopsies from or near the stoma or anastomosis may show mucosal erosion, which should not be used to evaluate for rejection
Focal crypt dropout should not be confused with crushing/squeezing artifact caused by biopsy procedure. Crushing artifact is not accompanied by increased numbers of lamina propria inflammatory cells or increased apoptotic activity in preserved crypts

Table 6.5 Severe ACR (Fig. 6.4)

Histologic features
Extensive crypt dropout
Extensive mucosal erosion and/or ulceration
Increased crypt apoptotic activity in areas adjacent to erosion/ulceration with residual crypts or in concurrent graft biopsies from other sites
Reactive and regenerative changes
Moderate to severe increase in the number of lamina propria inflammatory cells, usually extensive, consisting predominantly of mononuclear cells. Activated lymphocytes, eosinophils and neutrophils are usually present
Severe exfoliative rejection, a form of severe ACR, shows diffuse ulceration with neutrophilic exudates that involves the entire transplanted bowel
Differential diagnosis
Infectious enteritis, especially CMV enteritis with ulceration
Medication effect (see Sect. 6.1.4)
Chronic rejection, which can also show broad areas of ulceration, but will also show additional findings (see Sect. 6.2)
Potential diagnostic pitfalls
Biopsies from anastomotic site can show features of ulceration, which should not be used to evaluate for rejection

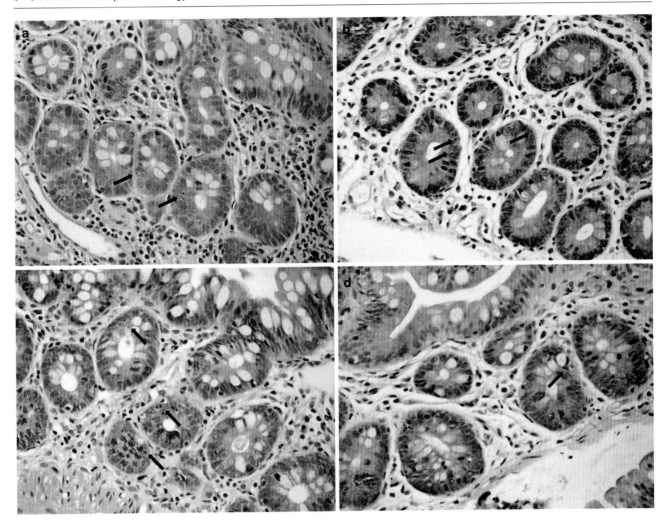

Fig. 6.1 (**a–d**) Examples of indeterminate for ACR. Minimally increased crypt apoptotic activity, <6 apoptotic bodies per 10 consecutive crypts, which does not meet the criteria for mild ACR. Note the differing morphologies of apoptotic bodies, which can be seen as small, pinpoint basophilic fragments of nuclear debris or as larger exploding nuclear fragments with a rim of clear cytoplasm (*arrows*, **a–d**)

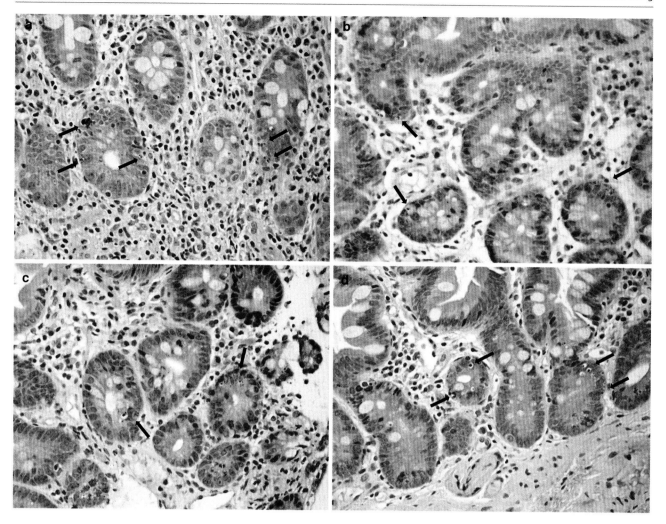

Fig. 6.2 (**a–d**) Examples of mild ACR. Mildly increased crypt apoptotic activity (*arrows*, **a–d**), ≥6 apoptotic bodies per 10 consecutive crypts, which is accompanied by epithelial reactive changes and increased lamina propria inflammatory cell infiltrates. No crypt dropout or erosion/ulceration is noted

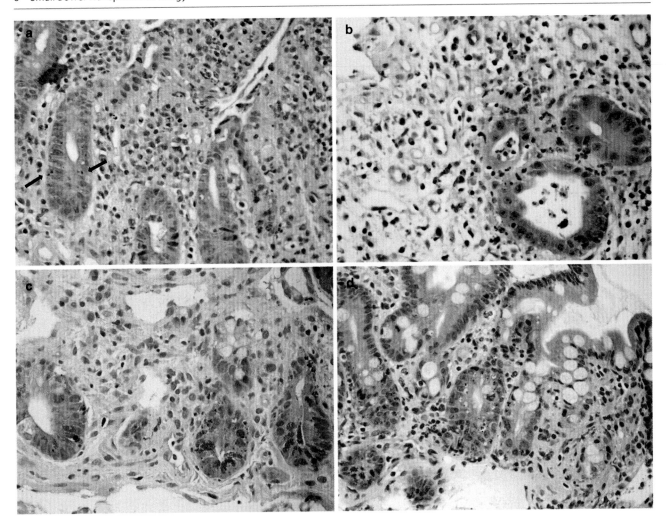

Fig. 6.3 (**a**–**d**) Examples of moderate ACR. In addition to increased crypt apoptotic activity (*arrows*, **a**), reactive epithelial changes, and increased lamina propria inflammatory cells, moderate ACR is further characterized by more severe mucosal injury including crypt dropout and withering (**a**), focal surface erosion (**b**), and confluent crypt apoptosis (**c**, **d**)

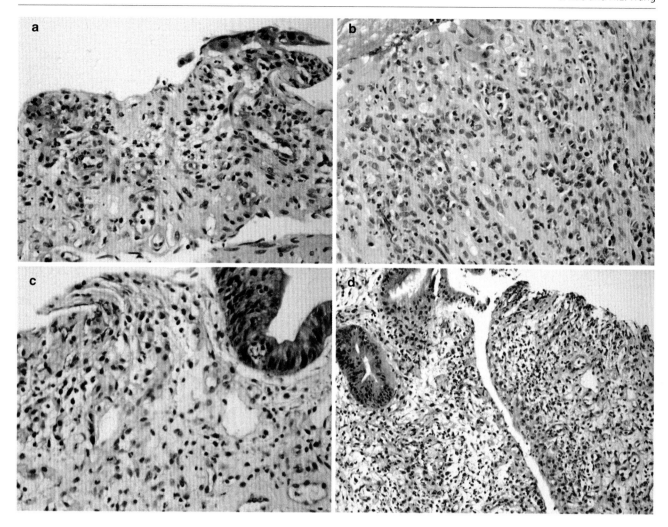

Fig. 6.4 (**a–d**) Examples of severe ACR. Extensive crypt dropout and ulceration are seen (**a, b**), with residual epithelial cells showing reactive and regenerative changes as well as increased apoptotic activity (**c, d**)

6.1.2 General Approach for Evaluation of Small Bowel Graft Biopsies

Routine H&E sections with multiple serial sections are examined.

Low-power examination

- Assess adequacy of biopsy: should be deep enough to include the entire mucosa and have at least ten well-oriented crypt bases (in specimens without crypt dropout or ulceration)
- Evaluate overall architecture
  - Intact: no ACR, IND, or mild ACR
  - Focal crypt dropout or focal erosion: possible moderate ACR
  - Extensive crypt dropout or ulceration: possible severe ACR

High-power examination

- Count crypt apoptotic bodies in crypt bases
  - May be challenging in tangentially sectioned biopsies, but crypt bases will generally contain Paneth cells
  - Apoptotic bodies seen in the surface epithelium should not be counted for the purpose of grading ACR
  - Choose the area with the highest apoptotic density to count
  - Search for confluent apoptosis, which may involve only a single or a few crypts
- Evaluate for viral inclusions and other infectious agents

6.1.3 Subclinical Rejection

Histological findings of ACR seen on surveillance/protocol biopsies in the absence of clinical symptoms, or subclinical rejection (SCR), is a relatively well-established entity in other solid organ transplants and has also been described in SBT [7]. SCR has been reported to account for 17–22 % of biopsies, with the majority showing findings of mild ACR. In their analysis, Takahashi et al. [7] demonstrated that SCR occurring within the first 3 months of transplantation was associated with decreased graft survival.

6.1.4 ACR and Its Differential from Medication Effect (Fig. 6.5)

Mycophenolate mofetil (CellCept) is a commonly used immunosuppressive medication following all types of organ transplantation, including SBT. Its use is limited primarily by gastrointestinal (GI) toxicity, which usually manifests as diarrhea. Recent studies have characterized the histological features of CellCept toxicity, which can affect the entire length of the GI tract and resemble graft-versus-host disease (GVHD), inflammatory bowel disease, acute self-limiting colitis, or ischemic colitis. Erosive or ulcerative enterocolitis can be seen [8–11]. Because increased crypt apoptotic activity is a key diagnostic feature for both ACR and CellCept toxicity (especially for CellCept toxicity with a GVHD-like pattern), differentiating between these two entities can be challenging. Clearly, correlation with the patient's medication history is essential in these situations. In addition, if concurrent biopsies are taken from native bowel (either small bowel or colon), the distribution of histological findings, in particular apoptotic bodies, can be used to help distinguish between ACR and CellCept toxicity. For example, if increased apoptotic bodies are seen in both graft and native bowel biopsies, this would favor CellCept toxicity because medication effect would be expected to affect both transplanted and native bowels. Conversely, if increased apoptotic bodies are seen only in graft biopsies but are not evident in native bowel biopsies, this would favor ACR because it would be expected to affect only transplanted bowel.

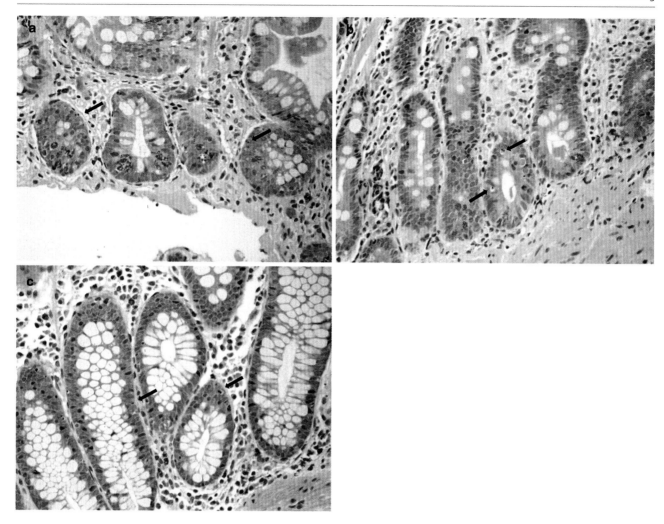

Fig. 6.5 (a–c) ACR and its differential from medication effect. This example shows increased apoptotic bodies (*arrows*) in a biopsy from the transplanted small bowel, which meets the diagnostic criteria for mild ACR (**a**). However, concurrent biopsies from native small bowel (**b**) and native colon (**c**) also show increased crypt apoptotic activity. The patient was confirmed to be on CellCept at the time of biopsies. The overall findings thus favored medication/CellCept effect over ACR

6.2   Chronic Rejection

Chronic rejection (Table 6.6 and Fig. 6.6) is a major cause of late graft dysfunction and loss, but it is difficult to diagnose both clinically and histologically on mucosal biopsies. Clinical suspicion for chronic rejection is raised in the presence of persistent diarrhea, nonhealing ulcers unresponsive to antirejection therapy, dysmotility, and poor nutritional status [12, 13]. The development of chronic rejection is often preceded by prior episodes of ACR. Increasing number of ACR episodes, occurrence of ACR within 30 days post transplantation and higher ACR grades all correlate with an increased risk of chronic rejection [12].

The resected graft specimen often shows extensive serosal adhesions. The bowel wall may be thickened, firm, and fibrotic-appearing. Localized strictures may be present owing to secondary ischemic injury. The mucosal folds may be flattened, and focal ulcers may be seen. The gross findings may resemble those seen for Crohn's enteritis.

Histologically, chronic rejection is defined by obliterative arteriopathy involving mesenteric, subserosal, muscularis propria, and submucosal vessels. This pathognomonic feature is more likely to be seen on a resected graft specimen than on mucosal biopsy. Some studies have attempted to identify potential mucosal changes associated with chronic rejection that may be recognizable on mucosal biopsy [12, 14], but consensus criteria have not been established yet. Because larger vessels are not typically sampled on mucosal biopsy, full-thickness biopsies have been suggested to allow for identification of diagnostic arterial changes.

To evaluate for chronic rejection, the following sections should be submitted from a graft resection specimen: areas of ulceration with adjacent nonulcerated mucosa, full-thickness of the bowel wall, subserosal and mesenteric vessels, and any grossly identified lesions such as stricture, mucosal nodules, serosal adhesions, among others.

Table 6.6 Chronic rejection (Fig. 6.6)

Histological features
Resected allograft specimens
Obliterative arteriopathy of subserosal, mesenteric, and less commonly, submucosal vessels, with intimal hyperplasia and luminal narrowing (eccentric or concentric narrowing)
Fibrosis of submucosa and subserosa, with possible fibrosis of lamina propria
Ulceration with widespread crypt loss
Crypt architectural distortion and pyloric metaplasia in regenerative areas
Extensive serosal adhesions with encasement of bowel loops in dense mesenteric fibrocollagenous tissue
Submucosal and myenteric neural hypertrophy
Mucosal changes possibly seen on biopsy
Pyloric metaplasia
Submucosal fibrosis
Patchy, mild fibrosis of lamina propria
Ulceration with neutrophilic exudates and granulation tissue
Distorted, blunted, and/or edematous villi
Widespread loss of crypts
Special studies
Trichrome-EVG stain to highlight intimal hyperplasia in arteries
Differential diagnosis
Treated ACR may show similar findings on mucosal biopsy, but persistence of these findings with pyloric metaplasia and persistent graft dysfunction are suggestive of evolving chronic rejection
Potential diagnostic pitfalls
Obliterative arteriopathy is the only defining feature of chronic rejection; thus, mesenteric vessels should be well sampled for graft resection specimens. In its absence, the constellation of other findings can be "consistent with" or "suggestive of" chronic rejection

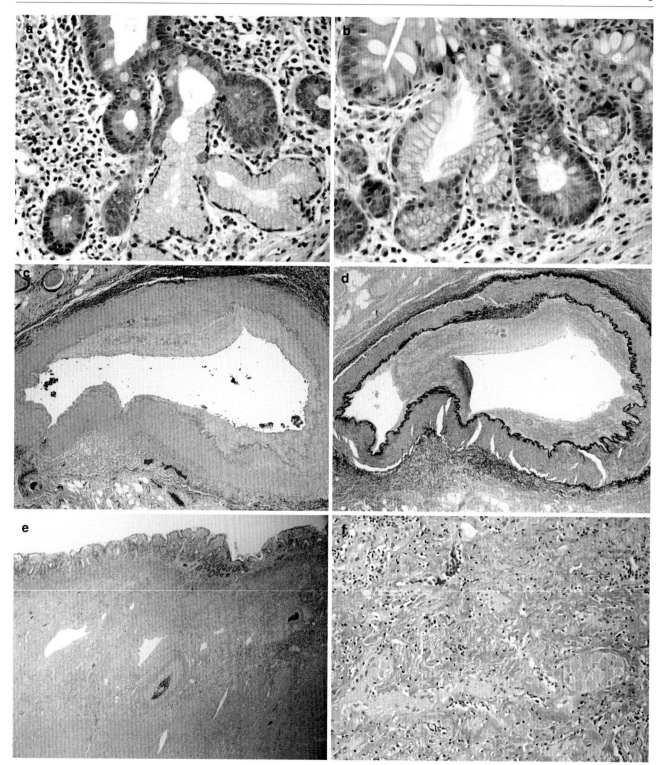

Fig. 6.6 (a–g) Examples of chronic rejection. Pyloric metaplasia is one of the features seen on graft biopsies that may suggest chronic rejection (a, b). Findings that can be seen on a graft resection specimen for chronic rejection include intimal hyperplasia with obliterative arteriopathy, which is the only diagnostic finding of chronic rejection of the small bowel transplants and most frequently involves mesenteric arteries (c, HE; d, EVG stain); submucosal fibrosis (e); submucosal neural hyperplasia (f). Obliterative arteriopathy can also be seen involving submucosal vessels (g)

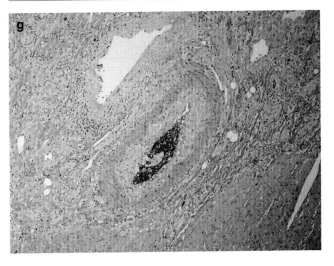

Fig. 6.6 (continued)

6.3 Antibody-Mediated Rejection

The contribution of antibody-mediated rejection (AMR) (Fig. 6.7) in SBT is not well characterized, and its frequency and clinical significance are uncertain. Although immunohistochemical staining for C4d has been used to evaluate for AMR in other solid organs, its use in SBT has not been found to be of clinical significance in few studies with a limited number of patients. In addition, C4d immunostaining does not appear to correlate with the presence of donor-specific antibodies or ACR in SBT patients [15, 16].

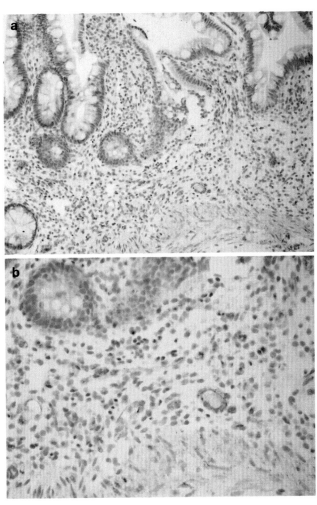

Fig. 6.7 (a, b) C4d immunostaining performed on a biopsy from transplanted small bowel. Positive staining in lamina propria capillary endothelial cells for C4d detected by immunohistochemistry, which is of uncertain significance in the management of SBT patients at this time. Additional studies in this area are needed

6.4   Infections

As a result of immunosuppression following SBT transplantation, infectious complications are a major source of patient morbidity and mortality (Tables 6.7, 6.8, and 6.9; Figs. 6.8, 6.9, and 6.10). Infectious etiologies can be bacterial, viral, fungal, and rarely, protozoal. Symptoms may include fever, diarrhea, and abdominal pain, which may overlap with symptoms seen for ACR. Correlation with cultures and serological studies is essential for the diagnosis and timely treatment with appropriate antimicrobial medications.

Table 6.7 Adenovirus enteritis (Fig. 6.8) [17, 18]

Incidence
Most common viral infection in SBT patients, affecting 24 % of pediatric patients in one study [17]
Patients generally present with increased ostomy output
Histological features
Typically infects enterocytes, which exhibit characteristic smudged nuclear chromatin, especially in the surface lining epithelium and not usually involving the crypts
Often show layering or "piling up" of the surface enterocyte nuclei
May be associated with a mildly increased lamina propria mixed inflammatory infiltrate and foci of active enteritis
Apoptosis is not prominent, but may involve the surface epithelium and superficial portion of the crypts, usually not involving the base of crypts like that seen for ACR
Special studies
Immunohistochemistry for adenovirus to highlight viral inclusions in the nuclei of infected enterocytes
Differential diagnosis
ACR, which would have more crypt apoptotic bodies and lack viral inclusions
Potential diagnostic pitfalls
When only rare viral inclusions are present, they can be easily overlooked on H&E sections. Routine immunohistochemical staining has been adopted by some institutions
Although simultaneous ACR may occur, it is difficult to assess its severity in the setting of adenovirus enteritis

Table 6.8 CMV enteritis (Fig. 6.9) [19–21]

Incidence
Greatly reduced owing to routine prophylactic antiviral therapy, currently reported to affect 1.5–5 % of SBT patients
Patients may present with increased ostomy output, GI bleeding, or rarely may be asymptomatic
Histological features
Typically infects endothelial and stromal cells in the lamina propria, but essentially any type of cell, such as epithelial and inflammatory cells, can be infected
Eosinophilic intranuclear and intracytoplasmic viral inclusions
A variable spectrum of inflammatory response ranging from no or minimal inflammation to deep ulceration. Typically, the mucosa shows neutrophil-rich infiltrates with cryptitis and crypt abscesses, accompanied by a varying degree of epithelial injury including increased apoptotic activity and crypt dropout
Occasional viral inclusions may persist after treatment
Special studies
Immunohistochemistry for CMV to highlight viral inclusions in infected cells
Differential diagnosis
ACR with or without ulceration, which would lack viral inclusions
Potential diagnostic pitfalls
In the setting of CMV enteritis, it is difficult to assess if there is concurrent ACR
In ulcerated areas, residual ganglion cells, degenerating cells, or reactive cells (such as macrophages and endothelial cells) could be mistaken as CMV-infected cells. Immunohistochemical staining for CMV is helpful in questionable cases

Table 6.9 Other potential causes of post-transplant infectious enteritis [4, 19]

Clinical
Rotavirus enteritis—causes diarrhea, which can be self-limited or protracted. Diagnosed with stool rotavirus antigen enzyme assay. Treated with supportive care
Cryptosporidium enteritis—seen rarely in post-SBT setting, may present with diarrhea or GI bleeding. Diagnosed on histology or stool culture. Treated with prolonged course of antimicrobials
Bacterial enteritis—including *C. difficile*, may present with diarrhea. Diagnosed with enzyme immunoassay for toxin A and B. Treated with antimicrobials
Histological features
Rotavirus enteritis—nonspecific, including mild-to-moderate villous blunting, increased lamina propria and intraepithelial inflammatory cells, surface epithelial disarray and piling up without viral inclusions
Cryptosporidium enteritis—characteristic 3–5 μm, spherical, basophilic trophozoites seen on the luminal border ("blue bead" appearance), mild villous blunting, typically no or little inflammatory response (Fig. 6.10)
Bacterial enteritis—ranging from minimal histological findings, active enteritis with or without ulceration, to pseudomembranous colitis
Differential diagnosis
Medication effect, which may show nonspecific histological findings. Correlation with drug history and laboratory findings is necessary

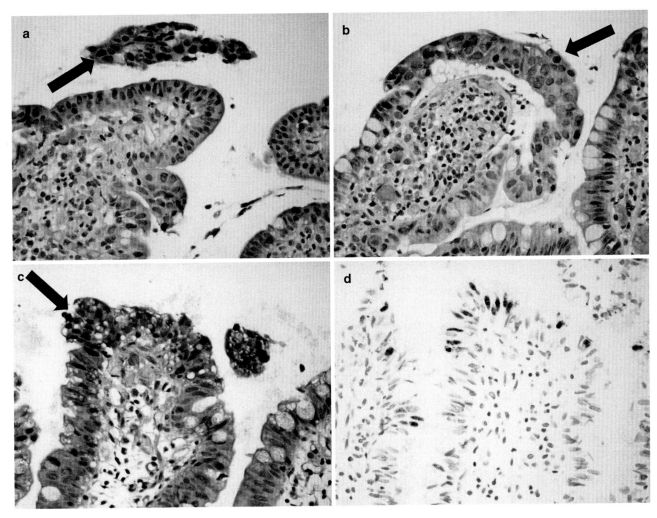

Fig. 6.8 (**a–d**) Adenovirus enteritis. Viral inclusions are typically seen in surface enterocytes, and appear as smudged, glassy nuclear chromatin. The infected enterocytes often become multilayered and pile up on each other (*arrows*, **a–c**). Immunohistochemistry for adenovirus confirms the presence of numerous infected epithelial cells (**d**, same case as **c**)

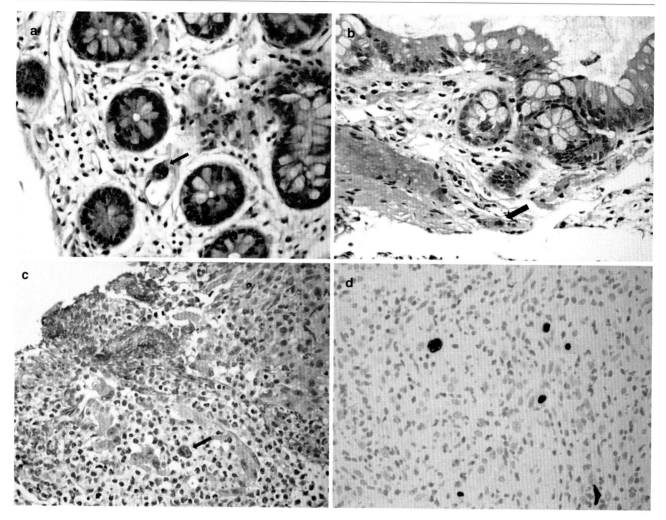

Fig. 6.9 (**a–d**) CMV enteritis. Eosinophilic CMV inclusions are seen in the nuclei as well as the cytoplasm of infected cells (*arrows*). The virus can infect various types of cells such as endothelial (**a**) and stromal (**b**) cells. In the examples shown in (**a, b**), there is no significant inflammatory response. More typically, CMV enteritis shows severely active inflammation with ulceration (**c**). Immunohistochemistry for CMV helps highlight multiple CMV-infected cells (**d**, same case as **c**)

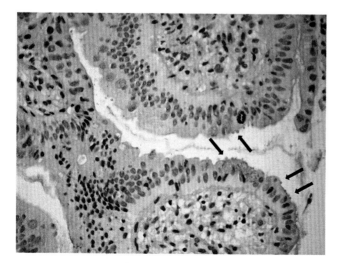

Fig. 6.10 *Cryptosporidium* infection (*arrows*) seen in a biopsy from transplanted small bowel, which has been reported in a small number of SBT cases

6.5 PTLD and Epstein-Barr Virus Infection
(Table 6.10; Fig. 6.11)

Although acute Epstein-Barr virus (EBV) infection is typically not a concern after transplantation, chronic infection with EBV in combination with immunosuppression can evolve into PTLD, which affects 10–13 % of SBT patients. PTLD can involve any body site, including the transplanted bowel, but often involves lymph nodes or other extraintestinal sites. The majority of post-SBT PTLD cases are EBV associated.

Table 6.10 Post-transplant lymphoproliferative disorder (Fig. 6.11) [22–24]

Incidence
10–13 % in SBT patients
Has been reported to affect the transplanted bowel in up to 71 % of cases
Majority of cases are EBV associated
Histological features
Proliferation of lymphoid cells with effacement of normal enteric architecture
Lymphoid infiltrates may be composed of a mixture of cells including small lymphocytes, large lymphocytes, immunoblasts, plasmacytoid cells, and plasma cells (polymorphic)
Alternatively, may be composed of a population of relatively uniform, usually large lymphocytes (monomorphic)
Special studies
In situ hybridization for EBV-encoded RNA (EBER)
Immunohistochemistry for lymphoid markers, including CD20, CD3, BCL2, CD138, kappa, lambda, among others
Flow cytometry analysis with demonstration of a monoclonal population
B- or T-cell gene rearrangement studies
Differential diagnosis
Benign reactive lymphoid aggregates, which are not uncommon in transplanted small bowel. They typically show normal follicular structures with germinal centers and do not efface or destroy the normal enteric architecture. Stains for EBER and selected lymphoid markers can be helpful in equivocal cases
Potential diagnostic pitfalls
Rare, scattered lymphocytes positive for EBER is not an uncommon finding in the post-transplant setting. This is not indicative of PTLD in the lack of appropriate histological findings
A minority of PTLD cases are not associated with EBV. EBER positivity is thus not required to make the diagnosis of PTLD

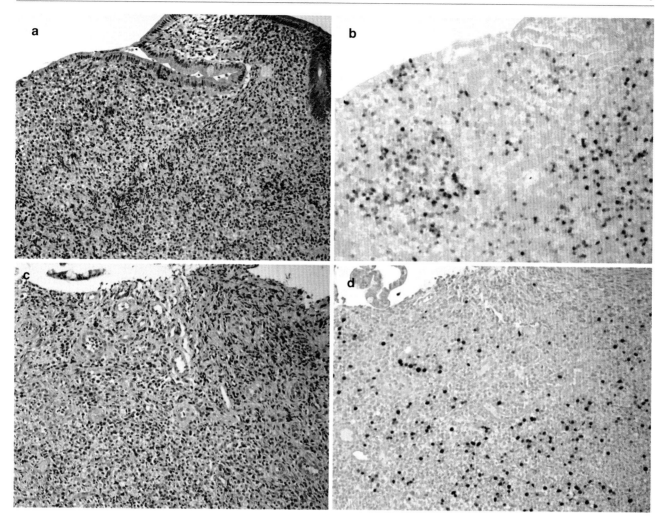

Fig. 6.11 (a–d) Examples of PTLD involving transplanted small bowel. Proliferation of lymphoid cells involving the mucosa with effacement of the normal architecture noted in a mucosal biopsy (**a**). The lymphoid cells showed diffuse positivity with immunohistochemistry for CD20 (*not shown*). EBER stain highlights numerous positive lymphoid cells (**b**). The lymphoid cells are of varying sizes and morphologies, consistent with polymorphous PTLD. Ulceration is noted in another example of polymorphous PTLD (**c**), which also shows numerous positive lymphoid cells on EBER stain (**d**)

References

1. Lee RG, Nakamura K, Tsamandas AC, Abu-Elmagd K, Furukawa H, Hutson WR, et al. Pathology of human intestinal transplantation. Gastroenterology. 1996;110:1820–34.
2. Smith JM, Skeans MA, Horslen SP, Edwards EB, Harper AM, Snyder JJ, et al. OPTN/SRTR 2013 annual data report: intestine. Am J Transplant. 2015;15 Suppl 2:1–16.
3. Smith JM, Skeans MA, Horslen SP, Edwards EB, Harper AM, Snyderf JJ, et al. OPTN/SRTR 2012 annual data report: intestine. Am J Transplant. 2014;14 Suppl 1:97–111.
4. Remotti H, Subramanian S, Martinez M, Kato T, Magid MS. Small-bowel allograft biopsies in the management of small-intestinal and multivisceral transplant recipients: histopathologic review and clinical correlations. Arch Pathol Lab Med. 2012;136:761–71.
5. Wu T, Abu-Elmagd K, Bond G, Nalesnik MA, Randhawa P, Demetris AJ. A schema for histologic grading of small intestine allograft acute rejection. Transplantation. 2003;75:1241–8.
6. Ruiz P, Bagni A, Brown R, Cortina G, Harpaz N, Magid MS, et al. Histological criteria for the identification of acute cellular rejection in human small bowel allografts: results of the pathology workshop at the VIII International Small Bowel Transplant Symposium. Transplant Proc. 2004;36:335–7.
7. Takahashi H, Kato T, Selvaggi G, Nishida S, Gaynor JJ, Delacruz V, et al. Subclinical rejection in the initial postoperative period in small intestinal transplantation: a negative influence on graft survival. Transplantation. 2007;84:689–96.
8. Delacruz V, Weppler D, Island E, Gonzalez M, Tryphonopoulos P, Moon J, et al. Mycophenolate mofetil-related gastrointestinal mucosal injury in multivisceral transplantation. Transplant Proc. 2010;42:82–4.
9. Nguyen T, Park JY, Scudiere JR, Montgomery E. Mycophenolic acid (CellCept and Myofortic) induced injury of the upper GI tract. Am J Surg Pathol. 2009;33:1355–63.
10. Parfitt JR, Jayakumar S, Driman DK. Mycophenolate mofetil-related gastrointestinal mucosal injury: variable injury patterns, including graft-versus-host disease-like changes. Am J Surg Pathol. 2008;32:1367–72.
11. Selbst MK, Ahrens WA, Robert ME, Friedman A, Proctor DD, Jain D. Spectrum of histologic changes in colonic biopsies in patients treated with mycophenolate mofetil. Mod Pathol. 2009;22:737–43.
12. Parizhskaya M, Redondo C, Demetris A, Jaffe R, Reyes J, Ruppert K, et al. Chronic rejection of small bowel grafts: pediatric and adult study of risk factors and morphologic progression. Pediatr Dev Pathol. 2003;6:240–50.
13. White FV, Ranganathan S. Small intestine. In: Liapis H, Wang HL, editors. Pathology of solid organ transplantation. Heidelberg: Springer; 2011. p. 347–70.
14. Swanson BJ, Talmon GA, Wisecarver JW, Grant WJ, Radio SJ. Histologic analysis of chronic rejection in small bowel transplantation: mucosal and vascular alterations. Transplantation. 2013;95:378–82.
15. de Serre NP, Canioni D, Lacaille F, Talbotec C, Dion D, Brousse N, et al. Evaluation of c4d deposition and circulating antibody in small bowel transplantation. Am J Transplant. 2008;8:1290–6.
16. Troxell ML, Higgins JP, Kambham N. Evaluation of C4d staining in liver and small intestine allografts. Arch Pathol Lab Med. 2006;130:1489–96.
17. Florescu DF, Islam MK, Mercer DF, Grant W, Langnas AN, Freifeld AG, et al. Adenovirus infections in pediatric small bowel transplant recipients. Transplantation. 2010;90:198–204.
18. Adeyi OA, Randhawa PA, Nalesnik MA, Ochoa ER, Abu-Elmagd KM, Demetris AJ, et al. Posttransplant adenoviral enteropathy in patients with small bowel transplantation. Arch Pathol Lab Med. 2008;132:703–5.
19. Ziring D, Tran R, Edelstein S, McDiarmid SV, Gajjar N, Cortina G, et al. Infectious enteritis after intestinal transplantation: incidence, timing, and outcome. Transplantation. 2005;79:702–9.
20. Guaraldi G, Cocchi S, Codeluppi M, Di Benedetto F, De Ruvo N, Masetti M, et al. Outcome, incidence, and timing of infectious complications in small bowel and multivisceral organ transplantation patients. Transplantation. 2005;80:1742–8.
21. Talmon GA. Histologic features of cytomegalovirus enteritis in small bowel allografts. Transplant Proc. 2010;42:2671–5.
22. Selvaggi G, Gaynor JJ, Moon J, Kato T, Thompson J, Nishida S, et al. Analysis of acute cellular rejection episodes in recipients of primary intestinal transplantation: a single center, 11-year experience. Am J Transplant. 2007;7:1249–57.
23. Abu-Elmagd KM, Mazariegos G, Costa G, Soltys K, Bond G, Sindhi R, et al. Lymphoproliferative disorders and de novo malignancies in intestinal and multivisceral recipients: improved outcomes with new outlooks. Transplantation. 2009;88:926–34.
24. Nassif S, Kaufman S, Vahdat S, Yazigi N, Kallakury B, Island E, et al. Clinicopathologic features of post-transplant lymphoproliferative disorders arising after pediatric small bowel transplant. Pediatr Transplant. 2013;17:765–73.

Vascularized Composite Tissue Transplant Pathology

7

Chandra Smart and Kourosh Beroukhim

Throughout the past few decades, vascularized composite tissue allotransplantation (CTA) has been introduced as an option for limb replacement and reconstruction of tissue defects. The first successful hand transplant was performed in Lyon, France, in September of 1998 [1]. Subsequently, over 90 upper extremity transplants have been performed, making these grafts the most common form of CTA [2]. These tissue grafts are complex in that they consist of a heterogeneous mixture of tissues, including skin, fat, muscle, nerves, lymph nodes, bone, cartilage, ligaments, and bone marrow [3]. In addition, they are unique because the skin provides a visual assessment of how the graft is functioning and aids in the diagnosis of rejection. The aforementioned phenomenon is secondary to the fact that the skin demonstrates the highest immunological activity in the context of acute rejection and is the first tissue to display signs of rejection [4]. Clinically, early cutaneous presentation allows immediate detection of acute rejection and is particularly essential given the absence of reliable serological or cellular markers indicative of composite tissue rejection [5].

The current classification system for the evaluation of CTA rejection was developed at the ninth Banff Allograft Pathology Meeting and grades the degree of rejection on a scale from 0 to 4. The diagnosis of rejection requires close communication with the clinician owing to the fact that some histological features we may see in "normal" skin biopsies may also be a harbinger of rejection in some of these transplant patients. Approximately 85 % of all hand allograft recipients have experienced at least one episode of acute skin rejection within the first year after transplant, and as many as 56 % have experienced multiple episodes [6]. These episodes may cause damage and loss of the graft. Therefore, it is of utmost importance to provide early and accurate diagnosis of rejection to prevent the aforementioned outcomes.

C. Smart, MD (✉)
Department of Pathology and Laboratory Medicine,
David Geffen School of Medicine at the University of California,
Los Angeles, CA, USA
e-mail: csmart@mednet.ucla.edu

K. Beroukhim, BS
David Geffen School of Medicine at the University of California,
Los Angeles, CA, USA

© Springer International Publishing Switzerland 2016
W.D. Wallace, B.V. Naini (eds.), *Practical Atlas of Transplant Pathology*, DOI 10.1007/978-3-319-23054-2_7

7.1 Acute Cellular Rejection and Differential Diagnosis

It is important to note that the histopathological diagnosis of rejection in CTA requires correlation with the clinical appearance of the skin. The clinical manifestations of rejection include mild, pink discoloration of the graft, erythema, macules progressing to red, infiltrated papules, edema, superficial erosion, necrosis, and onychomadesis [1, 7, 8]. Visual inspection together with histopathological evaluation of the skin is the gold standard in the diagnosis of skin rejection in vascularized composite allografts (VCA) [9]. According to the Banff 2007 Working Classification of Skin-containing Composite Tissue Allografts [10], visible skin changes should be reported as follows: no signs, less than 10 %, 10 % to 50 %, and greater than 50 %. The following histopathological descriptions are adapted from the Banff paper [10].

7.1.1 Grade 0

No or rare inflammatory infiltrates (Fig. 7.1)

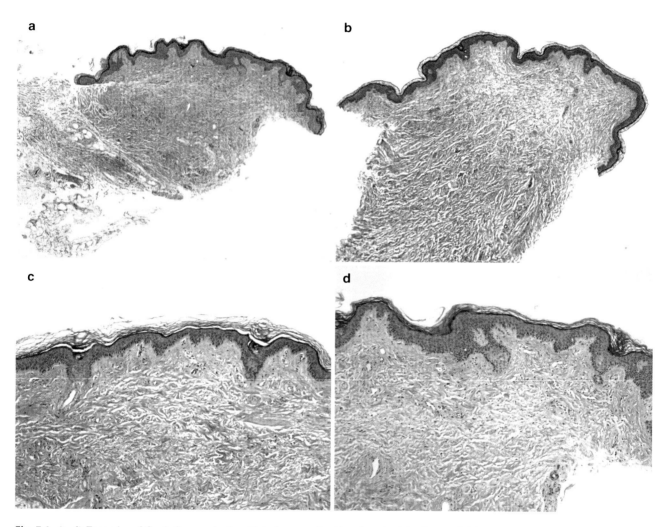

Fig. 7.1 (a–d) Examples of Grade 0—no rejection. Note the normal epidermis and minimal, superficial perivascular, lymphocyte-predominant inflammatory infiltrate

7.1.2 Grade I Rejection: Mild

The presence of mild inflammation characterizes mild, acute cellular rejection (ACR). There should be no involvement of the overlying epidermis (Figs. 7.2).

7.1.2.1 Differential Diagnosis

- Viral exanthem
- Drug eruption

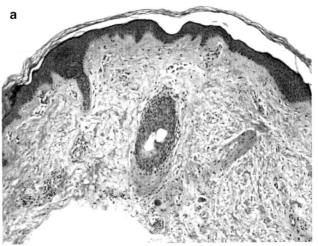

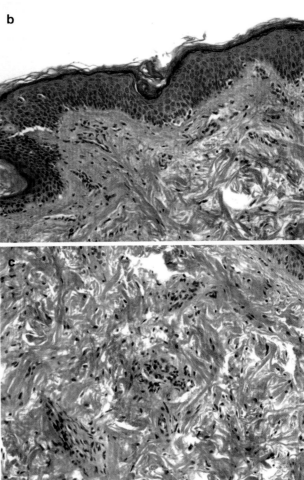

Fig. 7.2 (**a–c**) Examples of Grade I—mild rejection. Mild, superficial perivascular, lymphocyte-predominant inflammatory infiltrate. No epidermal involvement

7.1.3 Grade II Rejection: Moderate

The presence of a moderate to severe degree of perivascular inflammation, with or without mild epidermal and/or adnexal involvement (limited to spongiosis and exocytosis) without epidermal dyskeratosis/apoptosis characterizes moderate ACR (Fig. 7.3).

7.1.3.1 Differential Diagnosis

- Drug eruption
- Eczematous process (allergic/irritant contact dermatitis)
- Id reaction
- Infectious process (fungal, bacterial, viral)

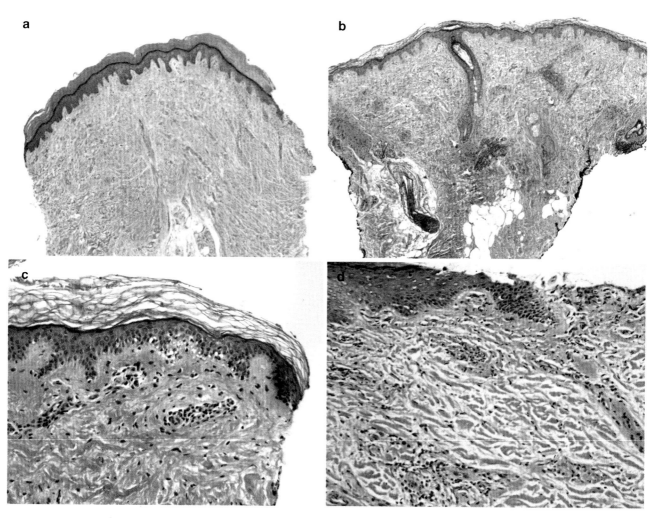

Fig. 7.3 (a–d) Examples of Grade II—moderate rejection. Moderate to severe perivascular inflammation with or without mild epidermal and/or adnexal involvement. Note the lymphocyte exocytosis into the epidermis without epidermal dyskeratosis/apoptosis (c). Note the epidermal spongiosis and lymphocyte exocytosis without epidermal dyskeratosis/apoptosis (d)

7.1.4 Grade III Rejection: Severe

The presence of dense inflammation and epidermal involvement with epithelial apoptosis, dyskeratosis, and/or keratinolysis characterizes severe ACR (Fig. 7.4).

7.1.4.1 Differential Diagnosis

- Drug eruption
- Eczematous process (allergic/irritant contact dermatitis)
- Infection

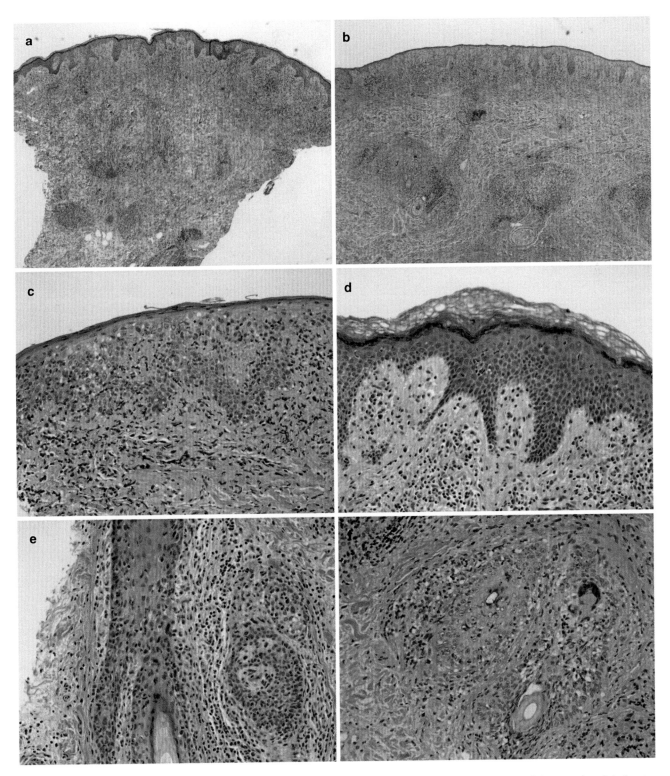

Fig. 7.4 (**a–f**) Examples of Grade III—severe rejection. Dense inflammation and epidermal involvement with epithelial apoptosis and dyskeratosis. Note the epithelial dyskeratosis/apoptosis involving the epidermis and the follicular epithelium (**c–f**)

7.1.5 Grade IV Rejection—Necrotizing Acute Rejection

Frank necrosis of the epidermis or other skin structures characterizes necrotizing acute rejection (Fig. 7.5).

7.1.5.1 Differential Diagnosis

- Drug eruption
- Infection

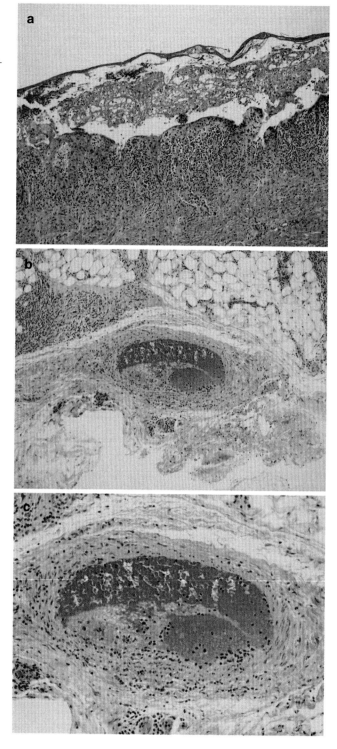

Fig. 7.5 (**a–c**) Examples of Grade IV—necrotizing rejection. Frank necrosis of the epidermis (**a**) or other skin structures and vasculitis (**b, c**)

7.2   Chronic Rejection

According to the Banff 2007 paper [10], insufficient data are available to define specific changes of chronic rejection. Chronic rejection has been defined by vasculopathy or atrophy and fibrosis of the skin and adnexal structures [11]. Other changes that may be seen include vascular narrowing, loss of adnexa, skin and muscle atrophy, fibrosis of deep tissue, myointimal proliferation, and nail changes [10]. It is important to note that the usual 4-mm punch biopsy may not be adequate in assessing graft vasculopathy and that a deeper tissue biopsy may be necessary to histologically document chronic rejection [12] (Fig. 7.6).

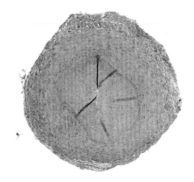

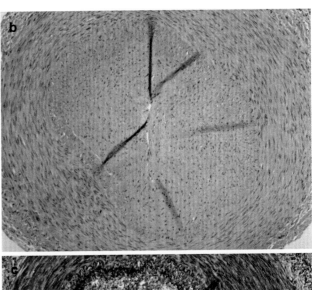

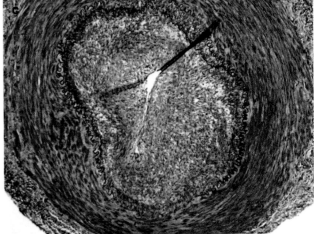

Fig. 7.6 (**a–c**) Chronic graft vasculopathy. Intimal hyperplasia with almost complete obliteration of the vascular lumen. Elastic Van Gieson (EVG) stain highlights the internal elastic lamina (**c**)

7.3 Antibody-Mediated Rejection

Capillary C4d complement deposition has been considered a marker of antibody-mediated rejection (AMR) and serves as a criterion for the pathological diagnosis of AMR in the Banff classification for solid organ transplantation [13]. Both immunohistochemical staining and direct immunofluorescence studies for C4d have aided in the diagnosis of AMR in solid organ transplantation. However, there has not yet been a consensus as to the role of routine C4d staining in composite tissue allografts to diagnose AMR [2].

References

1. Kanitakis J, Jullien D, Petruzzo P, Hakim N, Claudy A, Revillard JP, et al. Clinicopathologic features of graft rejection of the first human hand allograft. Transplantation. 2003;76:688–93.
2. Sarhane KA, Khalifian S, Ibrahim Z, Cooney DS, Hautz T, Lee WP, et al. Diagnosing skin rejection in vascularized composite allotransplantation: advances and challenges. Clin Transplant. 2014;28:277–85.
3. Siemionow M, Kulahci Y. Experimental models of composite tissue allograft transplants. Semin Plast Surg. 2007;21:205–12.
4. Lee WP, Yaremchuk MJ, Pan YC, Randolph MA, Tan CM, Weiland AJ. Relative antigenicity of components of a vascularized limb allograft. Plast Reconstr Surg. 1991;87:401–11.
5. Kanitakis J. The challenge of dermatopathological diagnosis of composite tissue allograft rejection: a review. J Cutan Pathol. 2008;35:738–44.
6. Petruzzo P, Lanzetta M, Dubernard JM, Landin L, Cavadas P, Margreiter R, et al. The international registry on hand and composite tissue allotransplantation. Transplantation. 2010; 90(12):1590–4
7. Cendales LC, Kirk AD, Moresi JM, Ruiz P, Kleiner DE. Composite tissue allotransplantation: classification of clinical acute skin rejection. Transplantation. 2006;81:418–22.
8. Lanzetta M, Petruzzo P, Dubernard JM, Margreiter R, Schuind F, Breidenbach W, et al. Second report (1998–2006) of the international registry of hand and composite tissue transplantation. Transpl Immunol. 2007;18:1–6.
9. Hautz T, Zelger BG, Weissenbacher A, Zelger B, Brandacher G, Landin L, et al. Standardizing skin biopsy sampling to assess rejection in vascularized composite allotransplantation. Clin Transplant. 2013;27:E81–90.
10. Cendales LC, Kanitakis J, Schneeberger S, Burns C, Ruiz P, Landin L, et al. The Banff 2007 working classification of skin-containing composite tissue allograft pathology. Am J Transplant. 2008;8:1396–400.
11. Schneeberger S, Ninkovic M, Piza-Katzer H, Gabl M, Hussl H, Rieger M, et al. Status 5 years after bilateral hand transplantation. Am J Transplant. 2006;6:834–41.
12. Kaufman CL, Ouseph R, Blair B, Kutz JE, Tsai TM, Scheker LR, et al. Graft vasculopathy in clinical hand transplantation. Am J Transplant. 2012;12:1004–16.
13. Mengel M, Sis B, Haas M, Colvin RB, Halloran PF, Racusen LC, et al. Banff 2011 meeting report: new concepts in antibody-mediated rejection. Am J Transplant. 2012;12:563–70.

Pancreas Transplant Pathology

Eric A. Swanson and Charles R. Lassman

Pancreas and simultaneous pancreas-kidney transplantation (SPK) are indicated for the treatment of type 1 diabetic patients, in particular, patients with diabetic nephropathy. Pancreas transplant alone may be indicated for type 1 diabetic patients with unstable "brittle diabetes" but no significant renal disease [1]. Pancreas transplantation is also infrequently performed to treat patients with type 2 diabetes. Diabetes mellitus and the sequelae of hyperglycemia is a major cause of end-stage renal disease, vascular disease, diabetic gastroparesis, neuropathy, and retinopathy. With a functional pancreatic graft, there is a stabilization of glucose levels and a decrease in the long-term consequences of hyperglycemia [2].

Pancreatic transplant was first performed in 1966 for endocrine dysfunction. Although at first graft survival was poor, over time, outcomes have progressively improved [3]. Initial surgical procedures involved whole graft transplant with polymer duct obliteration. Complications included vascular thrombosis, pancreatitis, and fistula formation. Bladder-drained grafts achieved an improved outcome, with the exocrine secretions drained into the bladder and insulin released to the venous system through the iliac veins. An advantage to this technique was the ability to monitor for rejection by quantification of exocrine enzymes such as amylase and lipase in the urine. Complications of this technique included hematuria, urine leak, urinary tract infection, and reflux pancreatitis. Another complication of this technique was

hyperinsulinemia, because insulin was directly released into the systemic circulation [4].

Most pancreatic transplants are now performed via pancreatic-duodenal transplantation [5]. The donor duodenum is anastomosed to the recipient small bowel or bladder. Venous drainage can be made to the portal system in these enteric-drained grafts, which is similar to the drainage of the native pancreas. There have been reports of lower complications with enteric-drained grafts, as well as fewer and less severe episodes of rejection [6].

Owing to the variation in major histocompatibility complex (MHC) expression in the various cellular components of the pancreas, acute cellular rejection (ACR) has been associated with damage to the exocrine function of the pancreas [7]. ACR preferentially affects the ducts, vessels, and acini. In contrast, antibody-mediated rejection (AMR) has been associated with hyperglycemia and islet injury, suggesting a vulnerability to microvascular injury and ischemia [8, 9].

Pancreatic allograft rejection is clinically asymptomatic, and detection relies on serum measurement of increased acinar enzymatic products such as amylase and lipase. Endocrine abnormalities in the form of hyperglycemia may also be noted in cases of severe rejection as well as in large vessel thrombosis and chronic rejection. Serum creatinine may also be used as a surrogate marker for pancreatic rejection in patients with SPK, although rejection is not always congruent between the two organs [10].

E.A. Swanson, MD (✉) • C.R. Lassman, MD, PhD
Department of Pathology and Laboratory Medicine, David Geffen School of Medicine at the University of California, Los Angeles, Los Angeles, CA, USA
e-mail: ericswanson1@gmail.com

© Springer International Publishing Switzerland 2016
W.D. Wallace, B.V. Naini (eds.), *Practical Atlas of Transplant Pathology*, DOI 10.1007/978-3-319-23054-2_8

8.1 Acute Cell-Mediated Rejection

The following are adapted from the Banff Schema for Grading Pancreas Allograft Rejection [11, 12] (Table 8.1).

8.1.1 Normal Pancreas

The normal pancreas shows absent to sparse inflammatory infiltrates, confined to the fibrous septa without involvement of septal structures. The fibrous septa are proportional to the size of the associated duct and vessels.

8.1.2 Indeterminate for Rejection

Focal active septal inflammation is present; however, the overall features do not fulfill the criteria for mild ACR

Table 8.1 Histological grading of ACR in pancreas transplant biopsies [11]

Category	Histology	Comments
Normal	Absent or inactive septal inflammation	Active inflammation includes blastic lymphocytes and/or eosinophils
Indeterminate for ACR	Active septal inflammation without additional findings	No ductitis or venulitis
Grade I/mild ACR	Active septal inflammation with ductitis or venulitis And/or 1–2 foci per lobule of acinar inflammation	Absent/minimal acinar injury
Grade II/moderate ACR	Minimal intimal arteritis (<25 % luminal compromise) And/or multiple foci (≥3 foci/lobule) of acinar inflammation with individual cell injury	No confluent or diffuse inflammation Requires differentiation from AMR
Grade III/severe ACR	Diffuse acinar inflammation with focal or diffuse confluent acinar cell necrosis And/or moderate to severe intimal arteritis And/or necrotizing arteritis	Requires differentiation from AMR

8.1.3 Grade I (Mild)

Active inflammation, including activated blastic lympho-cytes and/or eosinophils, involving septal structures is pres-ent. This inflammatory infiltrate may be variable. Foci of venulitis are seen, which is characterized by circumferential lymphocytic/inflammatory accumulation in the subendothe-lium with associated endothelial injury (Figs. 8.1 and 8.2). Ductal injury (ductitis) should also be present and will show lymphocytic or eosinophilic inflammation within the ductal epithelium. As a result of the inflammatory infiltrate, the ductal epithelial cells often show irregular spacing of the nuclei, anisonucleosis, and reactive changes (Fig. 8.3). Denudation of the epithelial cells may also be seen. The presence of venulitis or ductitis is sufficient for the diagnosis of mild ACR. In the absence of venulitis and ductitis, mild ACR may be diagnosed by the presence of focal acinar inflammation, limited to no more than two inflammatory foci per lobule with absent to minimal acinar cellular injury or dropout (Fig. 8.4).

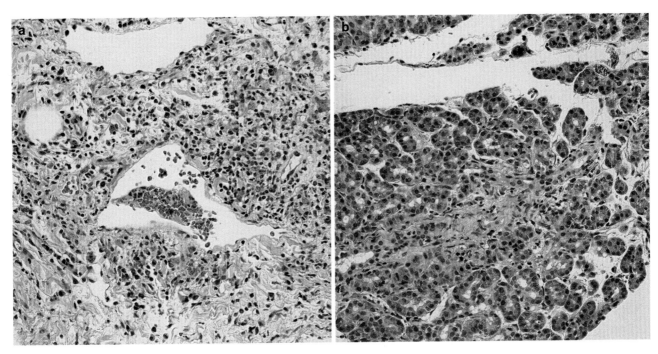

Fig. 8.1 (**a**, **b**) Mild ACR. (**a**) Interlobular septa show inflammation including activated blastic lymphocytes, plasma cells, eosinophils, and rare neutrophils. (**b**) The inflammatory infiltrate may be rich in eosinophils

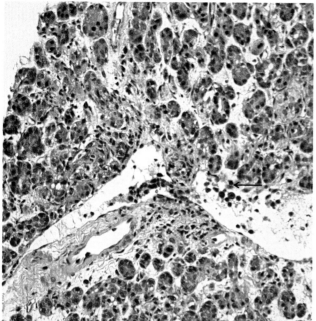

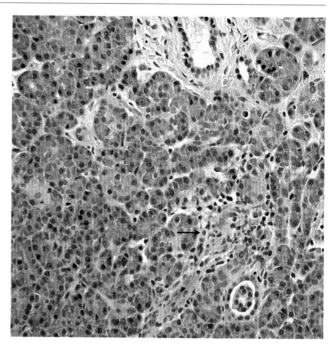

Fig. 8.2 Mild ACR. Septal vein shows venulitis with subendothelial accumulation of lymphocytes, activated blastic lymphocytes, and endothelial cell lifting and damage (*arrow*)

Fig. 8.4 Mild ACR. Spotty acinar inflammation and injury with minimal (*arrow*) to absent acinar dropout. These findings in isolation may also be diagnostic of mild ACR

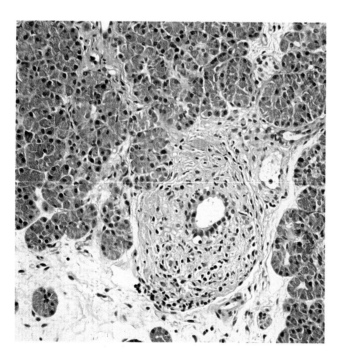

Fig. 8.3 Mild ACR. Interacinar duct with infiltration by lymphocytes and epithelial injury. The ductal epithelium shows cytoplasmic vacuolization, irregular nuclear spacing, and scattered apoptotic nuclei

8.1.4 Grade II (Moderate)

In addition to the histological findings of mild rejection, moderate ACR includes the finding of multifocal acinar inflammation (three or more foci per lobule) with individual acinar cell injury/dropout (Fig. 8.5). Alternatively, the diagnosis of moderate ACR may be defined by the presence of mild intimal arteritis, which is characterized by rare or occasional subendothelial inflammation by mononuclear cells without activation of or damage to the overlying arterial endothelium. The extent of the arteritis should compromise less than 25 % of the vessel lumen (Fig. 8.6).

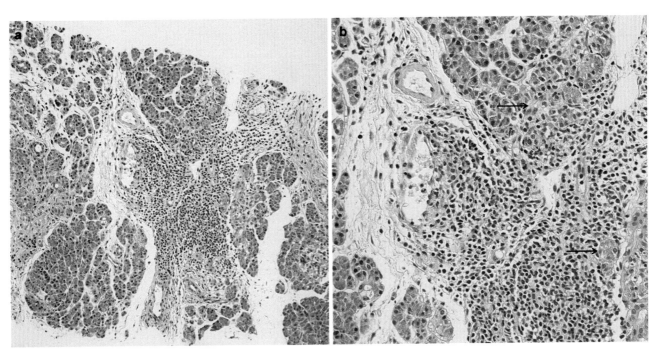

Fig. 8.5 (**a, b**) Moderate ACR. (**a**) Septal inflammation with lymphocytes, plasma cells, and rare eosinophils. (**b**) Focal acinar inflammation with spotty multifocal acinar injury/dropout (*arrows*). Septal venulitis is also identified

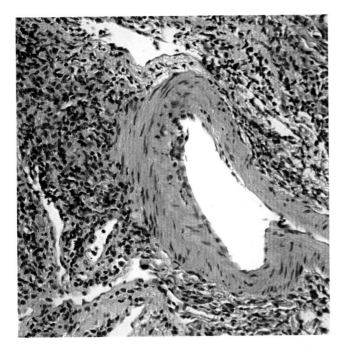

Fig. 8.6 Moderate ACR. Intimal arteritis with mononuclear cells in the subendothelium of this muscular artery. There is focal endothelial swelling and lifting/damage. The damage seen occupies less than 25 % of the arterial lumen

8.1.5 Grade III (Severe)

Severe ACR is characterized by diffuse acinar inflammation (confluent) with associated focal or diffuse confluent acinar cell necrosis. Interstitial edema and hemorrhage are characteristic of severe tissue damage. There should be no significant acinar tissue present without inflammatory infiltrate. Severe ACR may also be diagnosed by moderate to severe intimal arteritis, in which mononuclear cells are seen within the intima of a muscular artery with evidence of injury. This injury can manifest as endothelial cell activation or sloughing, margination of neutrophils, macrophage activation, proliferation of myofibroblasts within the intima, and fibrin leakage. Greater than 25 % of the vessel lumen should be compromised by the injury. Necrotizing arteritis, with focal or circumferential fibrinoid necrosis, may be seen with or without transmural inflammation. This finding can also be seen in AMR and should raise this possibility.

8.2 Antibody-Mediated Rejection

8.2.1 Hyperacute Rejection

This type of rejection is immediate graft rejection (within 1 h) due to preformed antibodies in the recipient serum. The histological findings include edema, acinar cell injury with vacuolization, degranulation, and spotty necrosis. Neutrophilic margination in capillaries and veins may be seen. In later stages, hemorrhagic necrosis is seen throughout the graft. Widespread fibrinoid vascular necrosis and thrombosis are present. C4d staining is seen throughout graft vasculature.

8.2.2 Accelerated AMR

Accelerated AMR is similar to hyperacute rejection, but occurs hours to days after transplantation.

8.2.3 Acute AMR

The diagnosis of acute AMR involves the combination of three criteria. These criteria include laboratory-confirmed circulating donor-specific antibodies (DSA), morphological evidence of tissue injury (see grading criteria later), and C4d positivity in interacinar capillaries (>5 % of acinar lobular surface) by immunostaining. When three of three criteria are met, the findings are diagnostic of AMR. If two of three criteria are met, the findings are consistent with AMR. If only one of three criteria is met, the finding requires exclusion of AMR. The grading of AMR is based on the histological features seen in the biopsy material (Table 8.2).

Table 8.2 Histological grading of AMR in pancreas transplant biopsies [12]

Category	Histology
Grade I/mild acute AMR	Well-preserved architecture
	Mild macrophage or mixed macrophage/neutrophilic infiltrates
	Rare acinar cell damage
Grade II/moderate acute AMR	Overall preserved architecture
	Interacinar macrophage or mixed macrophage/neutrophilic infiltrates
	Capillary dilation, capillaritis
	Congestion
	Multicellular acinar dropout
	Extravasated red blood cells
Grade III/severe acute AMR	Architectural disarray
	Scattered inflammatory infiltrates with interstitial hemorrhage
	Multifocal parenchymal necrosis
	Arterial and venous wall necrosis and thrombosis

8.2.4 Grade I/Mild Acute AMR

The pancreatic tissue shows well-preserved architecture. There are mild mononuclear and/or neutrophilic infiltrates with only rare acinar cell dropout/apoptosis (Fig. 8.7).

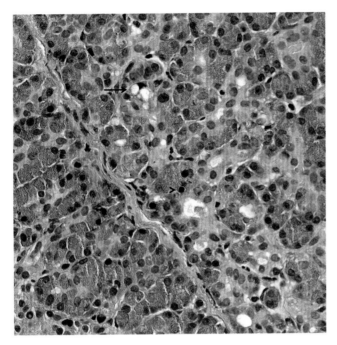

Fig. 8.7 Mild AMR. Subtle acinar cell injury with cytoplasmic swelling and vacuolization (*arrow*) and nuclear pyknosis/apoptosis (*arrowhead*)

8.2.5 Grade II/Moderate Acute AMR

There is overall preservation of pancreatic tissue architecture. Interacinar mononuclear, macrophage, and/or neutrophilic infiltrates are present. An immunostain for CD68 can highlight mononuclear infiltrate in cases without prominent neutrophils. See Table 8.2 for other histological features that may also be seen.

8.2.6 Grade III/Severe Acute AMR

The pancreatic tissue will show architectural disarray, with scattered inflammatory infiltrates in a background of interstitial hemorrhage.

8.2.7 C4d Staining Interpretation

C4d staining should be interpreted in interacinar capillaries. Immunohistochemical staining may be performed; however, immunofluorescence staining may be more sensitive. The staining pattern must be linear or granular. If the extent of lobular surface area is less than 5 %, the result is deemed negative. If there is staining of 5–50 % of the lobular surface area, the result is deemed focally positive (Fig. 8.8). If greater than 50 %, the result is deemed diffusely positive. Staining of the endothelium of larger arteries and veins, as well as septal and peripancreatic connective tissues is considered nonspecific staining.

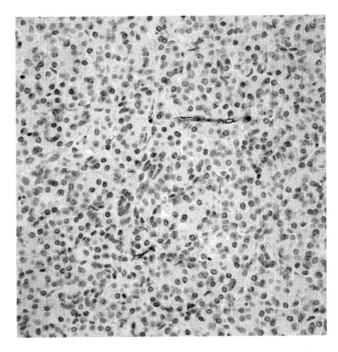

Fig. 8.8 AMR. Immunohistochemical staining for C4d shows focal positivity defined as between 5 and 50 % of the interacinar capillaries. In combination with the DSA studies as well as histological features, this may be supportive of AMR

8.3   Chronic Active AMR

Chronic active AMR is defined as the combination of features of AMR and chronic allograft rejection in the absence of acute T-cell–mediated rejection. Histological findings include arterial intimal fibrosis and infiltration of mononuclear cells with formation of a neointima.

8.4   Chronic Allograft Arteriopathy

Chronic allograft arteriopathy is characterized by arterial intimal fibrosis with mononuclear cell infiltration. Foam cell arteritis may also be seen (Figs. 8.9 and 8.10).

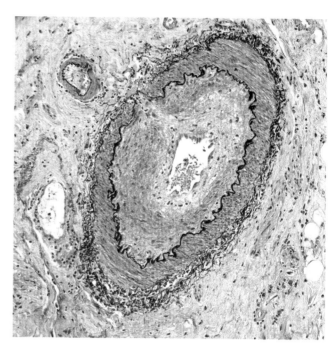

Fig. 8.9 Chronic allograft arteriopathy. Trichrome-elastin stain highlights arterial intimal fibrosis and neointima formation, with narrowing of the vessel lumen

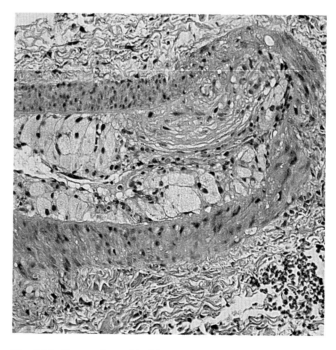

Fig. 8.10 Foam cell arteritis. Muscular artery with an intimal proliferation of fibroblasts and foamy macrophages. These findings may be seen in chronic allograft arteriopathy

8.5   Chronic Allograft Rejection/Graft Sclerosis

Staging of chronic rejection in pancreas transplant biopsies is based on the Banff Schema (Table 8.3) [11, 12].

8.5.1   Stage I (Mild Graft Fibrosis)

The pancreatic tissue shows mild expansion of fibrous septa. On biopsy, fibrosis occupies less than 30 % of the core surface. The acinar lobules show eroded and irregular contours; however, the central lobules are normal (Fig. 8.11).

Table 8.3 Histological staging of chronic rejection in pancreas transplant biopsies [11]

Category	Histology
Stage I (mild graft fibrosis)	Expansion of fibrous septa
	Acinar lobules show eroded, irregular contour
	Central lobules are normal
	Fibrosis <30 % of core surface
Stage II (moderate graft fibrosis)	Exocrine atrophy in the majority of lobules
	Acinar lobules show eroded, irregular contours
	Thin fibrous strands transverse individual acini
	Fibrosis occupies 30–60 % of core surface
Stage III (severe graft fibrosis)	Isolated residual acinar or islets present
	Fibrotic areas occupy >60 % of the core surface

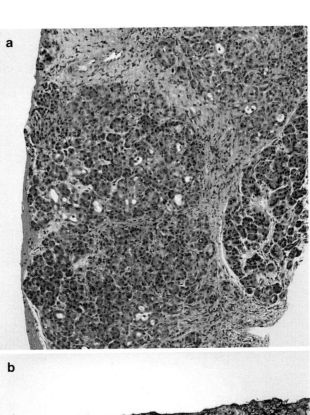

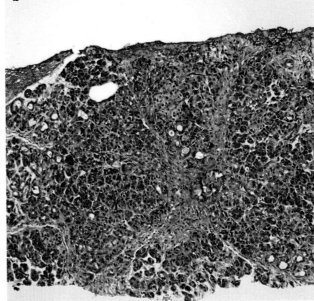

Fig. 8.11 (**a, b**) Stage 1 (mild) graft fibrosis. Subtle fibrous expansion of the septa and eroded, irregular contours of the acinar lobules. The central lobules remain without fibrosis. (H 200×) (**b**) Trichome stain highlights a mild increase in septal fibrosis as well as subtle fibrosis at the edge of the lobules, with sparing of the central lobules

8.5.2   Stage II (Moderate Graft Fibrosis)

There is moderate expansion of fibrous septa. On biopsy, fibrosis occupies 30–60 % of the core surface. Acinar lobules show exocrine atrophy with irregular contours involving most lobules. Central lobules show thin fibrous strands traversing individual acini (Fig. 8.12).

8.5.3   Stage III (Severe Graft Fibrosis)

Fibrosis is the predominant histological finding with involvement of greater than 60 % of the core surface. Only isolated residual acini or islets are present (Fig. 8.13).

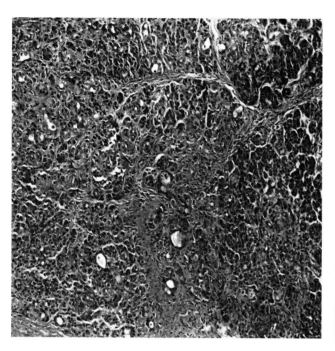

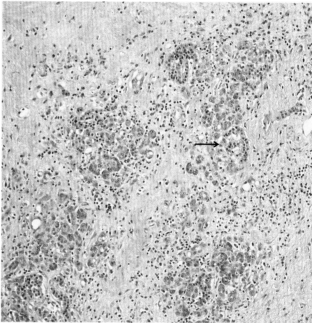

Fig. 8.12 Stage 2 (moderate) graft fibrosis. Trichrome-stained section shows moderate expansion of the fibrous septa with erosion of the contours of the lobules. Thin bands of fibrosis traverse the individual acini in both peripheral and central lobules. The patient was 10 years post pancreatic transplant

Fig. 8.13 Stage 3 (severe) graft fibrosis. There is severe graft fibrosis with atrophic acini and rare residual islets (*arrow*). The patient was 6 years post pancreatic transplant

8.6   Other Causes of Allograft Dysfunction

8.6.1   Ischemic Pancreatitis

Patients present with increased serum amylase and lipase or decreased urine amylase. Inflammation including foamy macrophages and neutrophils is seen within the pancreatic parenchyma. In mild disease, these findings are confined to the septa, but they may become diffuse in severe disease. Fat necrosis, edema, and coagulative necrosis can be seen.

8.6.2   Peripancreatitis

Patients present with systemic infectious symptoms and abdominal pain. Signs of peritonitis are seen. There may be peripancreatic fluid collections. Histologically, there is inflammation consisting of lymphocytes, plasma cells, eosinophils, and neutrophils present in the septa and at the periphery of lobules. The peripancreatic connective tissue may demonstrate necrosis and predominantly neutrophilic inflammation. Activated fibroblasts are seen with obliteration of septal structures and preservation of the center of the lobules (Fig. 8.14).

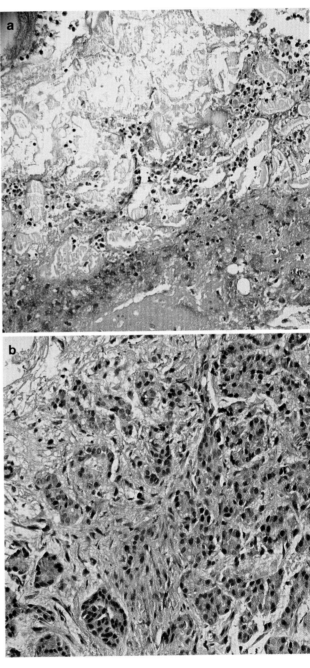

Fig. 8.14   (**a, b**) Peripancreatitis. (**a**) Acute inflammation and fat necrosis are seen in this graft biopsy. (**b**) The adjacent pancreatic tissue shows activation of fibroblasts and extension into the pancreatic parenchyma. This fibroblast proliferation should not be interpreted as chronic rejection

8.6.3 Infections

8.6.3.1 Cytomegalovirus Pancreatitis
Patients with cytomegalovirus (CMV) pancreatitis present with increased serum amylase and lipase. The tissue shows patchy mononuclear inflammation in septa and acini. The characteristic nuclear and cytoplasmic inclusions and cytomegaly are seen within infected acinar, endothelial, ductal, or stromal cells [13].

8.6.3.2 Bacterial or Fungal Infection
A variable inflammatory infiltrate composed of neutrophils, mononuclear cells, or granulomatous inflammation is seen. The inflammation is often necrotizing. Special stains may be performed to visualize the infectious organisms.

8.6.4 Recurrent Disease

8.6.4.1 Recurrent Autoimmune Disease (Diabetes Mellitus)
Recurrent autoimmune disease presents with hyperglycemia and/or islet cell autoantibodies (GAD-65, IA,2). There is islet-centered lymphocytic inflammation (isletitis) seen on biopsy tissue. In late stages, little to no inflammation is seen after beta cells have been destroyed [14].

References

1. Gruessner RW, Sutherland DE, Kandaswamy R, Gruessner AC. Over 500 solitary pancreas transplants in nonuremic patients with brittle diabetes mellitus. Transplantation. 2008;85:42–7.
2. Sudan D, Sudan R, Stratta R. Long-term outcome of simultaneous kidney-pancreas transplantation: analysis of 61 patients with more than 5 years follow-up. Transplantation. 2000;69:550–5.
3. Sutherland DE, Gruessner A. Long-term function (>5 years) of pancreas grafts from the international pancreas transplant registry database. Transplant Proc. 1995;27:2977–80.
4. Gaber AO, Shokouh-Amiri MH, Hathaway DK, Hammontree L, Kitabchi AE, Gaber LW, et al. Results of pancreas transplantation with portal venous and enteric drainage. Ann Surg. 1995;221:613–22.
5. Boggi U, Vistoli F, Egidi FM, Marchetti P, De Lio N, Perrone V, et al. Transplantation of the pancreas. Curr Diab Rep. 2012;12:568–79.
6. Nymann T, Hathaway DK, Shokouh-Amiri MH, Gaber LW, Abu-el-Ella K, Abdulkarim AB, et al. Patterns of acute rejection in portal-enteric versus systemic-bladder pancreas-kidney transplantation. Clin Transplant. 1998;12:175–83.
7. Steiniger B, Klempnauer J, Wonigeit K. Altered distribution of class I and class II MHC antigens during acute pancreas allograft rejection in the rat. Transplantation. 1985;40:234–9.
8. Melcher ML, Olson JL, Baxter-Lowe LA, Stock PG, Posselt AM. Antibody-mediated rejection of a pancreas allograft. Am J Transplant. 2006;6:423–8.
9. Nakhleh RE, Gruessner RW. Ischemia due to vascular rejection causes islet loss after pancreas transplantation. Transplant Proc. 1998;30:539–40.
10. Hawthorne WJ, Allen RD, Greenberg ML, Grierson JM, Earl MJ, Yung T, et al. Simultaneous pancreas and kidney transplant rejection: separate or synchronous events? Transplantation. 1997;63:352–8.
11. Drachenberg CB, Odorico J, Demetris AJ, Arend L, Bajema IM, Bruijn JA, et al. Banff schema for grading pancreas allograft rejection: working proposal by a multi-disciplinary international consensus panel. Am J Transplant. 2008;8:1237–49.
12. Drachenberg CB, Torrealba JR, Nankivell BJ, Rangel EB, Bajema IM, Kim DU, et al. Guidelines for the diagnosis of antibody-mediated rejection in pancreas allografts-updated Banff grading schema. Am J Transplant. 2011;11:1792–802.
13. Klassen DK, Drachenberg CB, Papadimitriou JC, Cangro CB, Fink JC, Bartlett ST, et al. CMV allograft pancreatitis: diagnosis, treatment, and histological features. Transplantation. 2000;69:1968–71.
14. Sutherland DE, Goetz FC, Sibley RK. Recurrence of disease in pancreas transplants. Diabetes. 1989;38 Suppl 1:85–7.

Post-transplantation Lymphoproliferative Disorders

Jonathan Said

Post-transplant lymphoproliferative disorders (PTLDs) comprise a wide spectrum of lymphoproliferative disorders that may be difficult to classify. They are potentially lethal, but clinical behavior is not always predictable from the histologic appearance. Factors that contribute to the development of PTLD include the type of transplant (solid organ versus bone marrow), degree of immunosuppression (which in turn generally relates to the type and duration of immunosuppressive therapy), HLA type, and viral status of the individual patient at the time of transplantation. Although the majority of cases of PTLDs are related to infection with the Epstein-Barr virus (EBV), there remains a subset of EBV-negative lymphomas that are less well-characterized. The spectrum of B-cell and N/K T-cell proliferations is illustrated from aggressive lymphomas to indolent localized EBV-related mucocutaneous ulcers.

9.1 Clinical Features of PTLDs

Early detection and prevention of PTLDs is an important strategy, particularly for younger high-risk patients who are negative for EBV exposure prior to transplant and require high levels of immunosuppression. Factors that predict the likelihood of developing PTLDs include younger age at time of transplantation, increased immunosuppression before developing EBV viremia, and higher peak EBV level [3]. In allogeneic hematopoietic stem-cell transplants, profound T-cell depletion of the allograft is a major risk factor for EBV-related PTLDs [4]. Adverse prognostic factors include older age, extranodal disease, and acute growth-versus-host disease (GVHD) [5]. Late-onset PTLDs, occurring 10 years or more following transplant, are seen most often in older

J. Said, MD
Department of Pathology and Laboratory Medicine,
David Geffen School of Medicine at the University of California,
Los Angeles, CA, USA
e-mail: jsaid@mednet.ucla.edu

male patients and tend to have a more aggressive clinical course.

9.2 Treatment of PTLDs

First-line therapy is usually initiated with reduction of immunosuppression, which may result in reduction or disappearance of PTLDs. In non-responding patients, chemotherapy, usually rituximab and CHOP (cyclophosphamide, hydroxy-daunorubicin, vincristine), is generally used [6]. Local therapy, including surgical resection and/or radiation, may apply to stage 1 disease, plasmacytoma-like PTLDs, and primary CNS PTLDs [7].

9.3 PTLDs Following Bone Marrow and Hematopoietic Stem-Cell Transplants

PTLDs following hematopoietic stem-cell transplant are invariably of donor origin. These usually occur soon after transplantation, 3 months or earlier. In addition to the more common types of PTLDs described below, cases of blastic plasmacytoid dendritic cell tumor have been described [8].

9.4 Differentiation of PTLDs from Rejection

Evaluating lymphoid and plasmacytic infiltrates in allograft biopsies for rejection versus PTLDs may be problematic, particularly in renal transplant core biopsies. Lesions of PTLDs are usually expansile and include cytologically abnormal cells, but differentiation from early lesions may be difficult. PTLDs usually do not contain acute inflammatory cells such as neutrophils and do not show other features of rejection such as endotheliitis or florid tubulitis, findings that are discussed elsewhere. It is possible for both processes to

© Springer International Publishing Switzerland 2016
W.D. Wallace, B.V. Naini (eds.), *Practical Atlas of Transplant Pathology*, DOI 10.1007/978-3-319-23054-2_9

occur in the same patient, and the diagnoses are not mutually exclusive. Immunohistochemical studies may be helpful because T cells usually predominate in rejection, and the infiltrates should contain few if any EBV-positive cells.

9.5   Classification of PTLDs

Although there are several classifications, they have been superseded by the classification published by the World Health Organization (WHO) in 2008 and shown in Table 9.1 [1]. There are three main categories: early lesions, polymorphic PTLDs, and monomorphic PTLDs. According to the WHO 2008 classification, low-grade lymphomas arising in transplant recipients are not considered specific subtypes of PTLDs and are generally not associated with EBV. However, rare cases of post-transplantation EBV–positive marginal zone lymphoma have been described that question this decision [2].

Table 9.1 Classification of PTLDs [1]

Early Lesions
Plasmacytic hyperplasia
Infectious mononucleosis-like
Polymorphic PTLDs
B-Cell Neoplasms:
Diffuse large B-cell lymphoma
Burkitt lymphoma
Plasma cell myeloma
Plasmacytoma-like lesions
T-Cell Neoplasms:
Peripheral T-cell lymphoma, NOS
Hepatosplenic T-cell lymphoma

While not entirely predictive of clinical behavior in the individual case, the WHO categories are broadly predictive of the course of the disease, particularly when correlated with molecular and clinical findings. Genetic studies have linked translocations (involving c-MYC, IgH, BCL2, and BCL6), mutations including PIM1 and PAX5, and other mechanisms that contribute to the aggressiveness of the disease. The tumor microenvironment may also influence the course of disease.

9.5.1   Early Lesions (Infectious Mononucleosis-Like PTLDs and Plasma Cell Hyperplasia)

Early lesions characteristically show retention of the architecture of involved tissues. Where lymph nodes are involved, the sinuses remain patent, and there is no extension beyond the capsule into adjacent tissues (Fig. 9.1). Reactive or

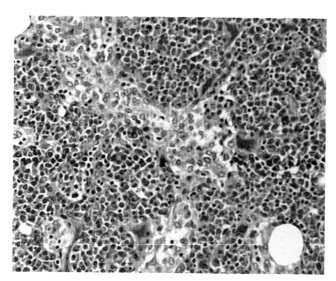

Fig. 9.1 Plasma cell hyperplasia. Section from a cervical lymph node biopsy showing retention of architecture with patent sinuses but uniform plasma cell proliferation. The cells are mature and lack cytologic abnormalities

hyperplastic germinal centers may be present. In plasma cell hyperplasia there are sheets of plasma cells but no architectural effacement (Fig. 9.2). Early lesions should be poly- or oligoclonal, and there should be no structural alterations in oncogenes or tumor suppressor genes. The adenotonsillar region is an important localization site for early lesions (Fig. 9.3), which tend to involve younger patients relatively soon after transplantation [9]. Patients with localized adenotonsillar PTLDs are more often females, and the outcome is generally favorable. PTLDs that resemble infectious mononucleosis are characterized by paracortical expansion (see Fig. 9.2) and a mixed population of lymphoid cells and plasma cells as well as immunoblasts, which may be numerous.

9.5.2 Polymorphic PTLDs

Polymorphic PTLDs (PL) include a broad spectrum of lymphoid proliferations with variable histologic appearance (Figs. 9.4, 9.5, 9.6, 9.7, 9.8, and 9.9). PL is frequently extranodal, including involvement of the gastrointestinal tract and the transplanted organ. The proliferations tend to occur relatively early after transplantation, overlapping with the early lesions. They may resolve with conservative therapy, but behavior is difficult to predict and dissemination may occur, including involvement of the central nervous system.

PL causes effacement of architecture by a proliferation that includes small lymphocytes, plasma cells, histiocytes, and variable numbers of transformed lymphoid cells and

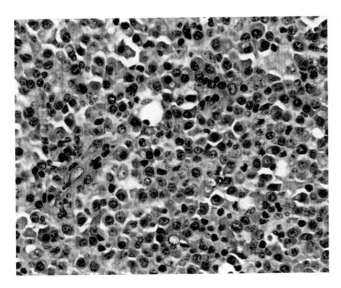

Fig. 9.2 Plasma cell hyperplasia. There are sheets of mature plasma cells lacking cytologic atypia

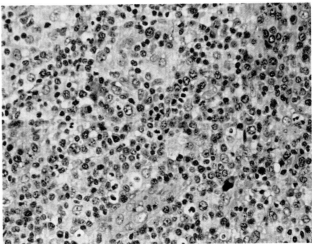

Fig. 9.4 Polymorphic PTLDs. There is a diffuse proliferation that includes small lymphocytes, histiocytes, plasma cells, and immunoblasts

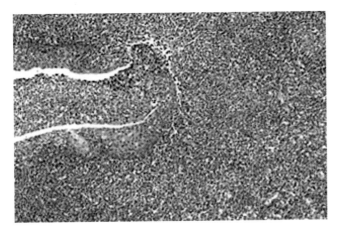

Fig. 9.3 Early PTLDs involving the tonsil. A tonsillar crypt is seen with sheets of small lymphoid cells and occasional immunoblasts in this form of early PTLDs that resembles infectious mononucleosis

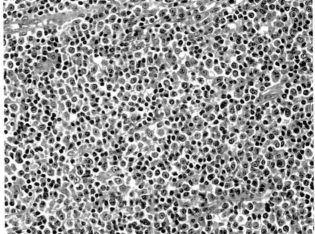

Fig. 9.5 Polymorphic PTLDs. This example is more cellular with sheet-like proliferation, but it retains the mixture of cell types, including plasma cells and immunoblasts

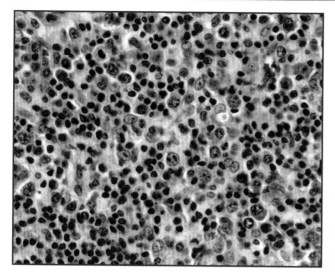

Fig. 9.6 Polymorphic PTLDs. In this example, in addition to scattered immunoblasts there is a mixed inflammatory background, including eosinophils

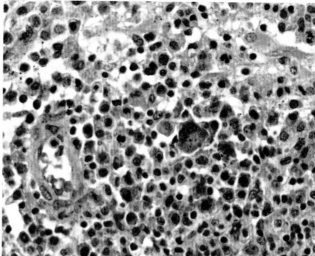

Fig. 9.8 Polymorphic PTLDs. In this example there are markedly dysplastic immunoblastic/plasmablastic cells as well as increased mitotic figures

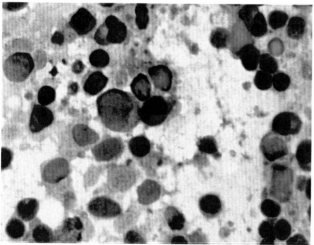

Fig. 9.7 Fine-needle aspirate from a case of polymorphic PTLDs. There is a spectrum of small- and intermediate-sized lymphoid cells as well as large immunoblasts in a background of "lymphoglandular" bodies

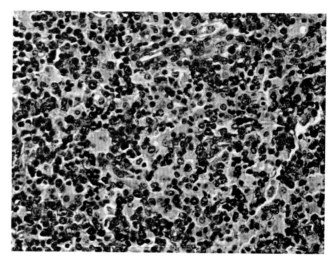

Fig. 9.9 Polymorphic PTLDs. Immunoblasts are evenly dispersed in a background that includes numerous reactive histiocytes

immunoblasts. There may be varying degrees of cytologic atypia, including the presence of Hodgkin and Reed Sternberg-like cells (Fig. 9.10). Areas of necrosis are frequently present. In addition to expression of EBV EBER, the large cells are often positive for EBV latent membrane protein (LMP1).

Despite the polymorphous appearance, PL is predominantly monoclonal in terms of immunoglobulin gene rearrangements and light-chain expression (Fig. 9.11) as well as EBV clonality, but lacks structural abnormalities in oncogenes or tumor suppressor genes. Mutations in the *BCL6* gene are sometimes found, although they lack *BCL6* rearrangement [10, 11].

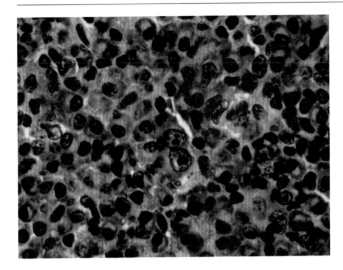

Fig. 9.10 Polymorphic PTLDs. Large immunoblasts resembling H/RS cells are seen

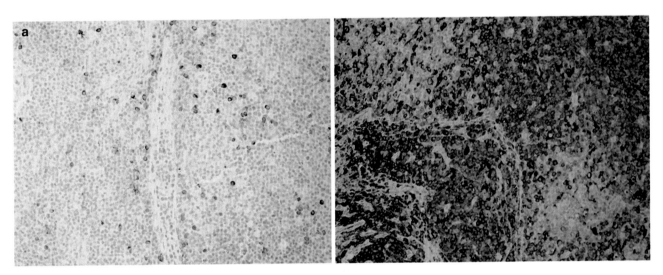

Fig. 9.11 Polymorphic PTLD stained for immunoglobulin light chain. Despite the polymorphic appearance, there is usually a light-chain restriction (in this case cytoplasmic staining for lambda light chain) in this form of PTLD. Kappa (**a**) and lambda (**b**) immunoperoxidase stains

9.5.3 Monomorphic PTLDs

Monomorphic PTLDs (ML) usually develop in older patients after a longer interval following transplantation. The lymphomas may be of B- or T-cell origin, and the T-cell types are described below. ML resembles aggressive forms of lymphoma encountered in the general, nontransplant population, particularly diffuse large B-cell lymphoma (DLBCL), and is classified according to the WHO [1]. It may present in lymph nodes and bone marrow as well as extranodal sites and may be disseminated involving the bone marrow. Different clones may be found at different sites of disease in the same patient with multifocal involvement. ML tends to have an aggressive course requiring systemic chemotherapy. It is composed of sheets of large malignant cells that may be centroblastic or immunoblastic in appearance (Figs. 9.12, 9.13, and 9.14). In addition to monoclonal immunoglobulin gene rearrangements, it often contains structural abnormalities in oncogenes or tumor suppressor genes, including *MYC*, *TP53*, and *RAS*.

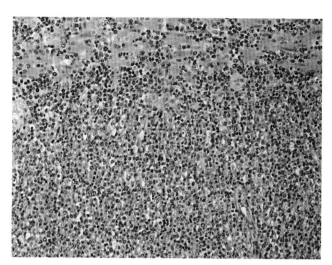

Fig. 9.12 Monomorphic PTLDs with features of diffuse large B-cell lymphoma. There are uniform large lymphoid cells infiltrating skeletal muscle in a soft-tissue mass

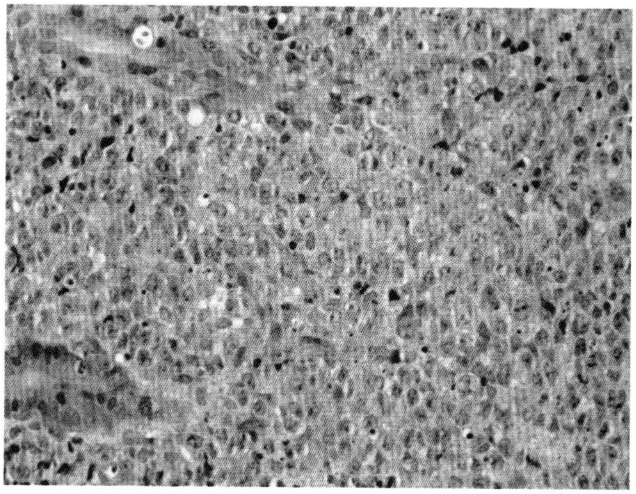

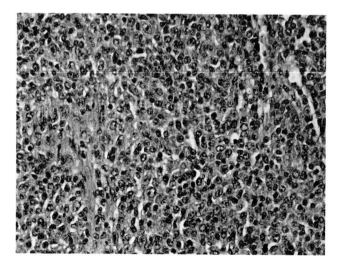

Fig. 9.13 Monomorphic PTLDs with features of diffuse large B-cell lymphoma. Higher power view reveals that most of the cells resemble centroblasts with round or oval nuclei and two or more evenly spaced nucleoli aligned at the nuclear membrane

Fig. 9.14 Monomorphic PTLDs with features of diffuse large B-cell lymphoma forming a mass in the wall of the colon. There are sheets of large centroblastic cells with frequent mitoses

9.5.4 Plasmablastic PTLDs

Plasmablastic PTLDs are an unusual form of monomorphic B-cell PTLDs. Most cases have been reported in male patients, and most are associated with EBV [12]. They are composed of sheets of blastic cells with prominent nucleoli and plasmacytoid cytoplasm (Fig. 9.15). They may express CD138 and be negative for CD20, and they are usually positive for EBV (Fig. 9.16). *MYC/IGH* rearrangements are seen in about one third of cases. Long-term remissions have been achieved, usually in combination with chemotherapy and reduced immunosuppression. Non–EBV-positive cases and those with cytogenetic abnormalities may have a worse prognosis.

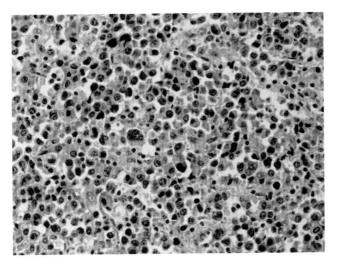

Fig. 9.15 Monomorphic PTLDs, plasmablastic. There are sheets of pleomorphic large cells with plasmablastic appearance and containing abundant amphophilic cytoplasm

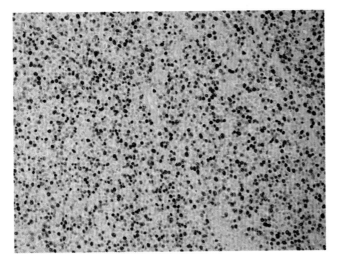

Fig. 9.16 Monomorphic PTLDs, plasmablastic. In-situ hybridization for EBV EBER reveals that most of the malignant cells are positive

9.5.5 Burkitt PTLD

Burkitt PTLD (BL) is a rare form of monomorphic PTLD. In the largest case series in adults, the median age at presentation was 38 years, predominantly males were affected, and the median interval following transplantation was 5.7 years [13]. The histology resembles Burkitt lymphoma in the immunocompetent population, with architectural effacement by sheets of cohesive or intermediate-sized blastic cells with round or oval nuclei and scant cytoplasm. Cytoplasmic vacuolization may be prominent in touch imprints. The cell population is uniform and homogeneous with few infiltrating inflammatory lymphocytes. There are numerous mitoses and evidence of high turnover in the form of tingible body or "starry sky" macrophages (Fig. 9.17). BL resembles endemic rather than sporadic cases in the expression of EBV, since almost all cases are positive (Fig. 9.18) [14]. BL is associated with translocations involving the *c-MYC* gene but lacks other molecular aberrations.

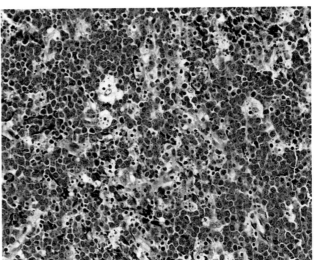

Fig. 9.17 Burkitt lymphoma. There are cohesive sheets of uniform intermediate-sized blasts admixed with numerous starry sky or tingible body macrophages. There are few infiltrating small lymphocytes

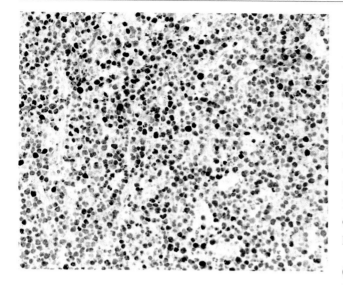

Fig. 9.18 Burkitt lymphoma with in-situ hybridization for EBV-EBER. The cells are uniformly positive

9.5.6 Plasmacytic PTLDs

Plasmacytic PTLDs present as monoclonal plasma cell proliferations similar to plasmacytomas associated with multiple myeloma. They are relatively uncommon, comprising about 4 % of cases of PTLDs [15]. The plasmacytoma lesions are usually extranodal and composed of sheets of plasma cells that are cohesive with very few small lymphocytes (Fig. 9.19). Dysplasia is variable, but blastic plasma cells as well as atypical and binucleated forms may be present. With immunohistochemistry there is expression of CD138 and lack of CD20 as well as cytoplasmic immunoglobulin light-chain restriction (Fig. 9.20). The median time from transplant is 3–4 years [15].

Clinically, patients usually present with extranodal tumors (including subcutaneous) that may be associated with monoclonal gammopathy. Unlike in conventional myeloma, the patients have normal calcium levels and only mild anemia. Association with EBV is variable (Fig. 9.21). Cases occurring in the pediatric age group are seen at a median time of 15 months after transplant and may resolve after minimal treatment. It has been suggested that cases of plasmacytic PTLDs not associated with EBV might represent a separate pathway for development of PTLDs [16].

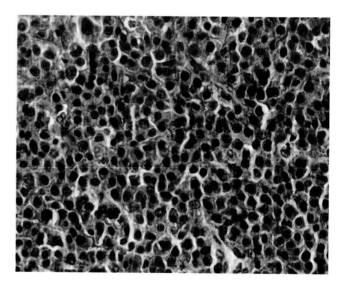

Fig. 9.19 PTLD resembling plasmacytoma. There are sheets of mature plasma cells with immunoglobulin light-chain restriction (immunostains not shown)

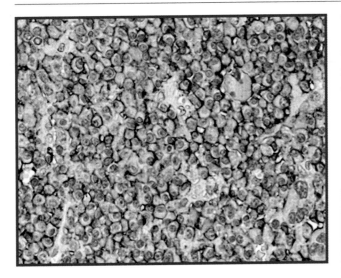

Fig. 9.20 PTLD resembling plasmacytoma. Immunostains are negative for CD20 but positive for CD138, shown here

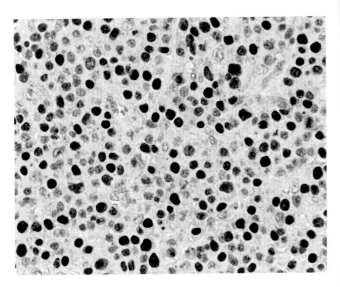

Fig. 9.21 PTLD resembling plasmacytoma. The neoplastic plasma cells are positive for EBV EBER with in-situ hybridization

9.5.7 Primary Central Nervous System PTLDs

Central nervous system presentation in PTLDs appears to represent a distinct clinicopathologic entity. It is has been described most commonly in renal transplant recipients and appears late with a median time of 54 months after transplant [6]. The tumors are mostly monomorphic and EBV-positive and about one third have deep brain involvement (Fig. 9.22). Therapies include methotrexate and brain radiation.

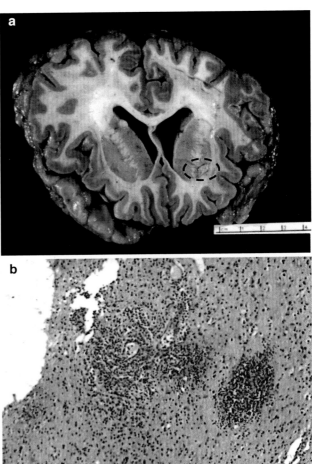

Fig. 9.22 PTLD of the central nervous system in a child developing soon after diagnosis of PTLD. (**a**), Section of the brain at autopsy reveals a partially necrotic deep-seated lesion (*circled*). (**b**), The neoplastic lymphoid infiltrate localized in relation to the vessels

9.5.8 EBV-Positive Mucocutaneous Ulcer: A Localized Indolent Form of PTLD

First described in 2011, mucocutaneous ulcer (MCU) is a rare indolent form of EBV-positive PTLD that presents with localized ulcers and resembles MCU in the general population [17]. MCU has been described in a variety of solid organ transplant patients, including renal, heart, and lung transplants. Although it can occur in patients as young as 19, most patients are older (sixth to seventh decade), with duration of immunosuppression up to 13 years. It presents with shallow ulcers in the oral mucosa or gastrointestinal tract, including the esophagus and small intestine, and the infiltrate is usually polymorphous in composition, including large B cells positive for CD20, CD30, and EBV EBER. Hodgkin and Reed-Sternberg-like cells are frequently encountered. Less commonly the lesions may comprise predominantly large cells resembling diffuse large B-cell lymphoma (DLBCL). The ulcers are sometimes undermined by a prominent inflammatory reaction [17]. It is important to recognize this form of PTLDs because it tends to remain localized and resolve with conservative therapy such as reduced immunosuppression or the administration of rituximab [17].

9.5.9 Hodgkin Lymphoma Type PTLD

Hodgkin lymphoma-type PTLDs (HL-PTLDs) are rare and typically occur in young patients (average age 30) but relatively later following transplantation. The histologic appearance resembles classical HL, with Hodgkin and Reed Sternberg cells (H/RS cells) in a mixed cellular background (Figs. 9.23 and 9.24). The phenotype resembles classical HL, including expression of CD15 and CD30 by the H/RS cells (Fig. 9.25), which are also positive both for EBV EBER and EBV-latent membrane protein (LMP1) (Fig. 9.26). The H/RS cells should have a limited expression of B-cell antigens, including CD20, CD79a, Pax5, OCT2, or BOB.1. Because of the presence of H/RS-like cells in other forms of PTLDs, particularly polymorphous PTLDs, the diagnosis of Hodgkin lymphoma following transplantation should be made with caution. The immunophenotype of the H/RS cells should be typical. EBV should be restricted to the H/RS cells and not expressed in the background population, which should not include EBV–infected lymphoid cells at various stages of transformation (Fig. 9.27).

HL-PTLDs may have an aggressive clinical course with a high rate of relapse following therapy and appear to be distinct clinicopathologic entities best treated with conventional HL therapy.

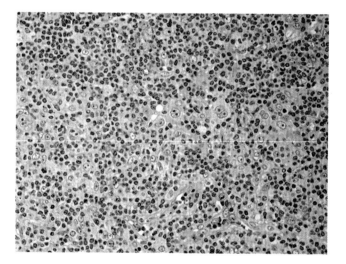

Fig. 9.23 Classic Hodgkin lymphoma (CHL) following transplantation. The features are typical of CHL, including the presence of Reed-Sternberg cells in a mixed background of lymphocytes, plasma cells, and histiocytes

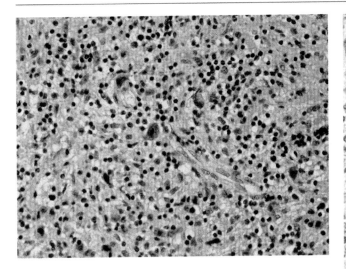

Fig. 9.24 Classic Hodgkin lymphoma arising in a mediastinal mass 5 years after a small bowel transplant. There are numerous H/RS cells in a mixed cellular background

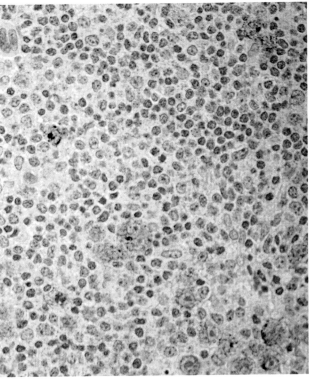

Fig. 9.26 Classic Hodgkin lymphoma (CHL) following transplantation. H/RS cells are positive for EBV-latent membrane protein (LMP1)

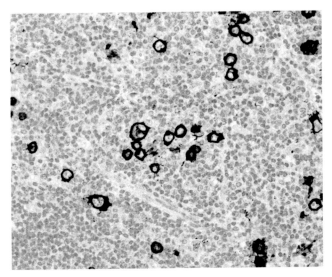

Fig. 9.25 Classic Hodgkin lymphoma (CHL) following transplantation. The H/RS cells have a typical phenotype, including staining for CD30

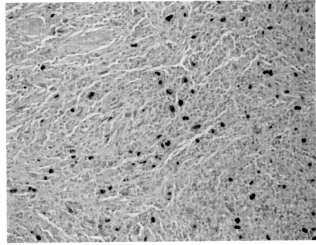

Fig. 9.27 Classic Hodgkin lymphoma PTLDs. EBV EBER in-situ hybridization shows that EBV is restricted to the H/RS cells

9.5.10 EBV-Negative PTLDs

Although the majority of lymphoid proliferations following transplant are EBV driven, about 20 % may be EBV-negative with pathogenetic mechanisms that are less well defined. These tend to occur in older patients with late onset after transplantation and include the majority of PTLDs of the T-cell type. In general they are less responsive to therapy and frequently aggressive. EBV-negative B-cell lymphomas are more often of germinal center origin and appear to be increasing in incidence [18–21].

9.5.11 T/NK-Cell PTLDs

T/NK-cell PTLDs (TL) affect all ages but usually develop in older male patients; they also occur late (median time of 72 months post-transplant). Most patients present with extranodal tumors [21]. T/NK cell PTLDs have been reported most frequently after kidney transplant, although organ-specific incidence is highest in heart transplant recipients. A variety of different T-cell lymphomas may be encountered and are classified according to the WHO [1]. Peripheral T-cell lymphoma not otherwise specified (PTCL, NOS) is most common and may have a variable appearance with admixed inflammatory cells, particularly macrophages (Figs. 9.28 and 9.29). In other cases there are sheets of large pleomorphic malignant cells (Fig. 9.30). Malignant cells are positive for T-cell markers such as CD3 (Fig. 9.31), although there may be loss of pan T-cell antigens, particularly CD7.

Less common types include hepatosplenic T-cell lymphoma, anaplastic large cell lymphoma, and angioimmunoblastic T-cell lymphoma [22]. T/NK cell large granular lymphocytic leukemia and anaplastic large-cell lymphoma have the best prognoses, whereas the other two behave poorly. About one third of cases are EBV-positive, and these may have a better survival rate, suggesting a different pathogenetic mechanism [21, 23].

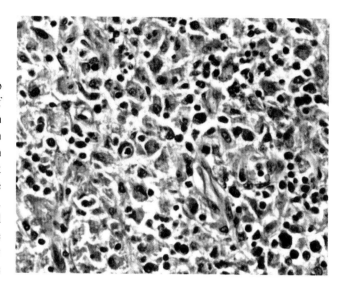

Fig. 9.29 Post-transplant peripheral T/NK cell lymphoma NOS. In this example, there are greater numbers of large markedly pleomorphic neoplastic cells in a histiocyte-rich background. Numerous apoptotic cells are present

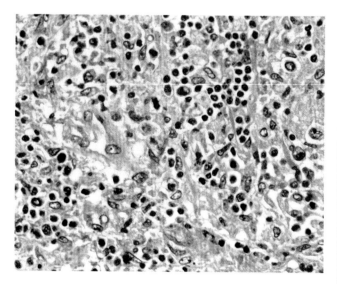

Fig. 9.28 Post-transplant peripheral T/NK cell lymphoma not otherwise specified (NOS). There are a spectrum of abnormal T cells, including large pleomorphic cells with prominent nucleoli in a background with small lymphocytes and histiocytes

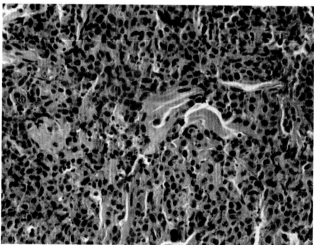

Fig. 9.30 Post-transplant peripheral T/NK cell lymphoma NOS. There are sheets of large malignant lymphoid cells in a sclerotic background

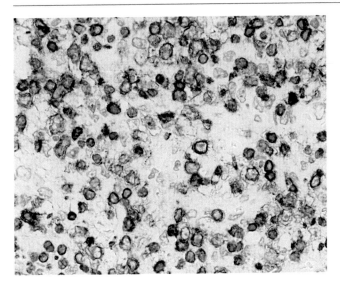

Fig. 9.31 Post-transplant peripheral T/NK cell lymphoma NOS. Large malignant cells stain positively for CD3

References

1. Swerdlow SH, Campo E, Harris NL, Jaffe ES, Pileri S, Stein H, et al., editors. WHO classification of tumours of haematopoietic and lymphoid tissues. Geneva: WHO Press; 2008.
2. Nassif S, Kaufman S, Vahdat S, Yazigi N, Kallakury B, Island E, et al. Clinicopathologic features of post-transplant lymphoproliferative disorders arising after pediatric small bowel transplant. Pediatr Transplant. 2013;17:765–73.
3. Weintraub L, Weiner C, Miloh T, Tomaino J, Joashi U, Benchimol C, et al. Identifying predictive factors for posttransplant lymphoproliferative disease in pediatric solid organ transplant recipients with Epstein-Barr virus viremia. J Pediatr Hematol Oncol. 2014;36:e481–6.
4. Rasche L, Kapp M, Einsele H, Mielke S. EBV-induced post transplant lymphoproliferative disorders: a persisting challenge in allogeneic hematopoetic SCT. Bone Marrow Transplant. 2014;49:163–7.
5. Styczynski J, Gil L, Tridello G, Ljungman P, Donnelly JP, van der Velden W, et al. Response to rituximab-based therapy and risk factor analysis in epstein barr virus-related lymphoproliferative disorder after hematopoietic stem cell transplant in children and adults: a study from the infectious diseases working party of the european group for blood and marrow transplantation. Clin Infect Dis. 2013;57:794–802.
6. Evens AM, David KA, Helenowski I, Nelson B, Kaufman D, Kircher SM, et al. Multicenter analysis of 80 solid organ transplantation recipients with post-transplantation lymphoproliferative disease: outcomes and prognostic factors in the modern era. J Clin Oncol. 2010;28:1038–46.
7. Zimmermann H, Trappe RU. EBV and posttransplantation lymphoproliferative disease: What to do? Hematology Am Soc Hematol Educ Program. 2013;2013:95–102.
8. Piccin A, Morello E, Svaldi M, Haferlach T, Facchetti F, Negri G, et al. Post-transplant lymphoproliferative disease of donor origin, following

haematopoietic stem cell transplantation in a patient with blastic plasmacytoid dendritic cell neoplasm. Hematol Oncol. 2012;30:210–3.
9. Khedmat H, Taheri S. Post-transplantation lymphoproliferative disorders localizing in the adenotonsillar region: report from the PTLD Int. Suvey. Ann Transplant. 2011;16:109–16.
10. Cesarman E, Chadburn A, Liu YF, Migliazza A, Dalla-Favera R, Knowles DM. BCL-6 gene mutations in posttransplantation lymphoproliferative disorders predict response to therapy and clinical outcome. Blood. 1998;92:2294–302.
11. Chadburn A, Chen JM, Hsu DT, Frizzera G, Cesarman E, Garrett TJ, et al. The morphologic and molecular genetic categories of posttransplantation lymphoproliferative disorders are clinically relevant. Cancer. 1998;82:1978–87.
12. Zimmermann H, Choquet S, Dierickx D, Dreyling MH, Moore J, Valentin A, et al. Early and late posttransplant lymphoproliferative disorder after lung transplantation--34 cases from the European PTLD Network. Transplantation. 2013;96:e18–9.
13. Zimmermann H, Reinke P, Neuhaus R, Lehmkuhl H, Oertel S, Atta J, et al. Burkitt post-transplantation lymphoma in adult solid organ transplant recipients: sequential immunochemotherapy with rituximab (R) followed by cyclophosphamide, doxorubicin, vincristine, and prednisone (CHOP) or R-CHOP, is safe and effective in an analysis of 8 patients. Cancer. 2012;118:4715–24.
14. Picarsic J, Jaffe R, Mazariegos G, Webber SA, Ellis D, Green MD, et al. Post-transplant Burkitt lymphoma is a more aggressive and distinct form of post-transplant lymphoproliferative disorder. Cancer. 2011;117:4540–50.
15. Karuturi M, Shah N, Frank D, Fasan O, Reshef R, Ahya VN, et al. Plasmacytic post-transplant lymphoproliferative disorder: a case series of nine patients. Transpl Int. 2013;26:616–22.
16. Nalesnik MA. Plasma cell tumors in transplant patients. Blood. 2013;121:1247–9.
17. Hart M, Thakral B, Yohe S, Balfour Jr HH, Singh C, Spears M, et al. EBV-positive mucocutaneous ulcer in organ transplant recipients: a localized indolent posttransplant lymphoproliferative disorder. Am J Surg Pathol. 2014;38:1522–9.
18. Johnson LR, Nalesnik MA, Swerdlow SH. Impact of Epstein-Barr virus in monomorphic B-cell posttransplant lymphoproliferative disorders: a histogenetic study. Am J Surg Pathol. 2006;30:1604–12.
19. Nelson BP, Nalesnik MA, Bahler DW, Locker J, Fung JJ, Swerdlow SH. Epstein-Barr virus-negative post-transplant lymphoproliferative disorders: a distinct entity? Am J Surg Pathol. 2000;24:375–85.
20. Craig FE, Johnson LR, Harvey SA, Nalesnik MA, Luo JH, Bhattacharya SD, et al. Gene expression profiling of Epstein-Barr virus-positive and -negative monomorphic B-cell posttransplant lymphoproliferative disorders. Diagn Mol Pathol. 2007;16:158–68.
21. Herreman A, Dierickx D, Morscio J, Camps J, Bittoun E, Verhoef G, et al. Clinicopathological characteristics of posttransplant lymphoproliferative disorders of T-cell origin: single-center series of nine cases and meta-analysis of 147 reported cases. Leuk Lymphoma. 2013;54:2190–9.
22. Kraus TS, Twist CJ, Tan BT. Angioimmunoblastic T cell lymphoma: an unusual presentation of posttransplant lymphoproliferative disorder in a pediatric patient. Acta Haematol. 2014;131:95–101.
23. Tiede C, Maecker-Kolhoff B, Klein C, Kreipe H, Hussein K. Risk factors and prognosis in T-cell posttransplantation lymphoproliferative diseases: reevaluation of 163 cases. Transplantation. 2013;95:479–88.

Appendix

Transplant Biopsy Templates

Heart

Cardiac Transplant Biopsy Evaluation [1, 2]

Endomyocardium (Biopsies):

Grade of Acute Cell-Mediated Rejection
- **Grade 0 R: No evidence of cell-mediated rejection.**
- **Grade 1 R, mild:** Interstitial and/or perivascular infiltrate with up to 1 focus of myocyte injury.
  - Previous Grade 1A: Perivascular infiltrates without myocyte injury.
  - Previous Grade 1B: Sparse interstitial infiltrates without myocyte injury.
- **Grade 2 R, moderate**: Two or more foci of infiltrate with associated myocyte damage.
  - Previous Grade 3A: Multifocal prominent infiltrates and/or myocyte injury.
- **Grade 3 R, severe:** Diffuse infiltrate with multifocal myocyte damage $\pm$ edema $\pm$ hemorrhage $\pm$ vasculitis
  - Previous Grade 3B: Diffuse infiltrates with myocyte injury.
  - Previous Grade 4: Diffuse polymorphous infiltrate with myocyte injury $\pm$ hemorrhage $\pm$ edema $\pm$ vasculitis.

Grade of Antibody-Mediated Rejection (AMR/Humoral Rejection)
- **pAMR 0: Negative for antibody mediated rejection.**
- **pAMR 1 (H+):** Histologic features of AMR alone
- **pAMR 1 (I+):** Immunopathologic features of AMR alone
- **pAMR 2:** Pathologic AMR—both H and I positive
- **pAMR 3:** Severe pathologic AMR—hemorrhage, edema, acute inflammation

(Immunofluorescence and immunoperoxidase studies reported separately)

Additional Findings
- Suboptimal biopsy: only _____ fragments of endomyocardium
- Quilty effect (A): Endocardium only.
- Quilty effect (B): With myocyte encroachment (myocyte injury may be present).
- Ischemic changes (A): Up to 6 weeks post-transplant.
- Ischemic changes (B): Late; >6 weeks post-transplant.
- Infection present: Rejection not interpretable.
- Lymphoproliferative disorder.
- Biopsy site present.
- Epicardial adipose tissue present.
- Other.

Comments
_____was notified of the preliminary diagnoses at _____ on _____.

© Springer International Publishing Switzerland 2016
W.D. Wallace, B.V. Naini (eds.), *Practical Atlas of Transplant Pathology*, DOI 10.1007/978-3-319-23054-2

References

1. Stewart S, Winters GL, Fishbein MC, Tazelaar HD, Kobashigawa J, Abrams J, et al. Revision of the 1990 working formulation for the standardization of nomenclature in the diagnosis of heart rejection. J Heart Lung Transplant. 2005;24:1710–20.
2. Berry GJ, Angelini A, Burke MM, Bruneval P, Fishbein MC, Hammond E, et al. The ISHLT working formulation for pathologic diagnosis of antibody-mediated rejection in heart transplantation: evolution and current status (2005–2011). J Heart Lung Transplant. 2011;30:601–11.

Lung

Lung Transplant Evaluation [1]
(Transbronchial Biopsies):

Acute rejection

None	**Grade A0** (no perivascular inflammatory infiltrates)
Minimal	**Grade A1** (scattered, infrequent perivascular mononuclear infiltrates in alveolated lung parenchyma **with no/few eosinophils and no endothelialitis**)
Mild	**Grade A2** (more frequent perivascular mononuclear infiltrates surrounding venules and arterioles, ± eosinophils and endothelialitis)
Moderate	**Grade A3** (extension of the inflammatory cell infiltrate into perivascular and peribronchiolar alveolar septa)
Severe	**Grade A4** (diffuse perivascular, interstitial and air-space infiltrates of mononuclear cells with prominent alveolar pneumocyte damage and endothelialitis)

Airway inflammation ("R" denotes revised grade from 1996 scheme)

None	**Grade B0** (no significant inflammation)
Low grade	**Grade B1R** (mononuclear cells within the sub-mucosa)
High grade	**Grade B2R** (epithelial damage with necrosis or metaplasia and marked intra-epithelial lymphocytic infiltration)
Ungradeable	**Grade BX** (no airway or obscured by infection or artifact)

Airway fibrosis (Histologic correlate of BOS—evaluated with Trichrome/EVG stain)
Present, mild/moderate/severe
Absent

Special staining
Acid-fast (AFB) stain (positive/negative) for organisms
Methenamine silver (GMS) stain (positive/negative) for organisms

Other
Suboptimal specimen consisting of____fragments of alveolar tissue
Capillary neutrophilia (may indicate antibody-mediated process) [2]
Aspiration pneumonia
Acute pneumonia
Organizing pneumonia
Acute lung injury (with diffuse alveolar damage)
Acute alveolar hemorrhage
Alveolar hemosiderosis (common s/p transplantation)

Comment:
The case was discussed with _____ at _____ on _____.

References

1. Stewart S, Fishbein MC, Snell GI, Berry GJ, Boehler A, Burke MM, et al. Revision of the 1996 working formulation for the standardization of nomenclature in the diagnosis of lung rejection. J Heart Lung Transplant. 2007;26:1229–42.
2. Berry G, Burke M, Andersen C, Angelini A, Bruneval P, Calabrese F, et al. Pathology of pulmonary antibody-mediated rejection: 2012 update from the Pathology Council of the ISHLT. J Heart Lung Transplant. 2013;32:14–21.

Kidney

Kidney, Transplant [1–3] (Needle Core Biopsy)

Acute tubular injury (acute tubular necrosis)

Acute antibody-mediated changes with C4d staining of peritubular capillaries, consistent with acute/active antibody-mediated rejection (*correlation with donor-specific antibodies is required for definitive diagnosis of antibody-mediated rejection*)

FOCAL C4d staining of peritubular capillaries with mild peritubular capillaritis (*correlation with donor-specific antibodies is required for definitive diagnosis of antibody-mediated rejection*)

At least moderate capillary inflammation WITHOUT C4d deposition, suggestive of C4d-negative antibody-mediated rejection (*correlation with donor-specific antibodies is required for definitive diagnosis of antibody-mediated rejection*)

C4d deposition without morphologic evidence of active rejection

Not diagnostic of antibody-mediated rejection (C4d negative and insufficient morphologic evidence of antibody-mediated rejection)

Borderline changes
"Suspicious" for acute T-cell–mediated rejection

Acute cell-mediated rejection
IA. Tubulointerstitial type
IB. Tubulointerstitial type with severe tubulitis (>10 lymphocytes/ tubular cross section)
IIA. Vascular type
IIB. Vascular type with severe intimal arteritis comprising >25 % of the luminal area
III. Transmural arteritis and/or arterial fibrinoid necrosis of medial smooth muscle cells with lymphocytic inflammation

Negative for acute cell-mediated rejection

Features suggestive of resolving acute cell-mediated rejection (see comment)

Cannot evaluate for acute cell-mediated rejection (see comment)

Chronic active T-cell-mediated rejection
(Chronic transplant arteriopathy)

Chronic transplant glomerulopathy (early/mild)
(The presence of C4d deposition strongly suggests this process is **chronic active antibody-mediated rejection**)
(In the absence of C4d deposition, this process may be **inactive chronic AMR or chronic active C4d-negative AMR**)

Interstitial fibrosis and tubular atrophy
 I. Mild interstitial fibrosis and tubular atrophy (<25 % of cortical area)
 II. Moderate interstitial fibrosis and tubular atrophy (26–50 % of cortical area)
 III. Severe interstitial fibrosis and tubular atrophy/ loss (>50 % of cortical area)

No significant chronic tubulointerstitial changes

Thrombotic microangiopathy (see comment)

Features suggestive of thrombotic microangiopathy (see comment)

BK virus nephropathy

Arteriolar medial hyalinosis, suggestive of chronic calcineurin inhibitor toxicity

Other:

Comment:
The preliminary diagnosis of this STAT prepared biopsy was "" and was discussed with the renal transplant team on ____.
The preliminary diagnosis of this ROUTINE biopsy was "" and was discussed with the renal transplant team on ____.
The presence of tubulitis without significant associated interstitial inflammation is suggestive of treated/resolving acute cell-mediated rejection.
In the setting of BK virus nephropathy, acute cell-mediated rejection cannot be reliably determined.
The primary differential diagnosis for the etiology of thrombotic microangiopathy in the setting of renal transplant is AMR-associated thrombosis versus calcineurin inhibitor-induced thrombosis. Other considerations include: TTP, HUS, malignant hypertension, scleroderma renal crisis, and other drug toxicity.

Microscopic Exam Synoptic

The specimen for conventional light microscopy is studied with hematoxylin and eosin, periodic acid-Schiff, periodic acid-methenamine silver (Jones), and Masson's trichrome stained sections.

The specimen consists of:
Cores:____
Composition: cortex, medulla, corticomedullary junction
Number of glomeruli (completely sclerotic): ____
Number of arteries:____

Acute Changes
  Glomeruli
    Allograft glomerulitis score:
    g0 – No glomerulitis
    g1 – Glomerulitis in <26 % of glomeruli
    g2 – Glomerulitis in 26–50 % of glomeruli
    g3 – Glomerulitis in >50 % of glomeruli
    N/A

  Tubulointerstitium
    Tubulitis score:
    t0 – No or rare mononuclear cells in tubules
    t1 – Foci with 1–4 cells/tubular cross section
    t2 – Foci with 5–10 cells/tubular cross section
    t3 – Foci with >10 cells/tubular cross section

    Interstitial inflammation score:
    i0 – No significant inflammation
    i1 – 10–25 % parenchyma inflamed
    i2 – 26–50 % parenchyma inflamed
    i3 – >50 % parenchyma inflamed

  Vessels
    Intimal arteritis score:
    v0 – No arteritis
    v1 – Mild-to-moderate intimal arteritis
    v2 – Severe intimal arteritis comprising >25 % of the luminal area
    v3 – Transmural arteritis and/or arterial fibrinoid necrosis of medial smooth muscle cells
    N/A

    Peritubular capillaritis score:
    ptc 0 – No significant cortical ptc, or <10 % of PTCs with inflammation
    ptc 1 – Greater than or equal to 10 % of cortical peritubular capillaries with capillaritis, with 3–4 luminal inflammatory cells

ptc 2 – Greater than or equal to 10 % of cortical peritubular capillaries with capillaritis, with 5–10 luminal inflammatory cells

ptc 3 – Greater than or equal to 10 % of cortical peritubular capillaries with capillaritis, with >10 luminal inflammatory cells

Chronic Changes
Glomeruli
Allograft glomerulopathy score:

cg0 – No GBM double contours by light microscopy or EM

cg1a – No GBM double contours by light microscopy but GBM double contours (incomplete or circumferential) in at least three glomerular capillaries by EM with associated endothelial swelling and/or subendothelial electron-lucent widening

cg1b – One or more glomerular capillaries with GBM double contours in ≥ 1 nonsclerotic glomerulus by light microscopy; EM confirmation is recommended if EM is available

N/A

Mesangial matrix expansion score:

mm0 – No increase

mm1 – ≤ 25 of nonsclerotic glomeruli have moderate matrix increase

mm2 – 26–50 % of nonsclerotic glomeruli have moderate matrix increase

mm3 – >50 % of nonsclerotic glomeruli have moderate matrix increase

N/A

Tubulointerstitium
Tubular atrophy score:

ct0 – Minimal atrophy

ct1 – Mild atrophy less than or equal to 25 % tubules

ct2 – Moderate atrophy 26–50 % tubules

ct3 – Severe atrophy >50 % tubules

Interstitial fibrosis score:

ci0 – Minimal fibrosis less than or equal to 5 %

ci1 – Mild fibrosis less than or equal to 25 %

ci2 – Moderate fibrosis 26–50 %

ci3 – Severe fibrosis >50 %

Vessels
Arterial fibrous intimal thickening score:

cv0 – No chronic vascular changes

cv1 – Less than or equal to 25 % vascular narrowing intimal fibrosis ± internal elastic lamina disruption, intimal foam cells

cv2 – 26–50 % vascular narrowing intimal fibrosis ± internal elastic lamina disruption, intimal foam cells

cv3 – >50 % vascular narrowing intimal fibrosis ± internal elastic lamina disruption, intimal foam cells

N/A

Arteriolar hyalinosis thickening:

ah0 – No insudative lesions in the media

ah1 – Mild hyaline thickening in the media of at least one arteriole

ah2 – Moderate hyaline thickening in the media of at least one arteriole

ah3 – Severe hyaline thickening in the media of at least one arteriole

N/A

Immunofluorescence Microscopy

Immunofluorescence microscopy is performed on frozen sections stained with hematoxylin and eosin, periodic acid-Schiff, and fluoresceinated antisera to human IgG, IgA, IgM, C1q, C3, C4d, albumin, fibrinogen, and kappa and lambda immunoglobulin light chains.

Immunofluorescence microscopy is performed on frozen sections stained with hematoxylin and eosin, periodic acid-Schiff, and fluoresceinated antisera to human fibrinogen and C4d.

Each frozen section consists of:
Composition: cortex, medulla, corticomedullary junction
Number of glomeruli (completely sclerotic):_____

Fibrinogen staining: Nonspecific/Arteriolar/Glomerular

Scoring of C4d staining:
    C4d0: Negative: 0 %
    C4d1: Minimal C4d staining: <10 %
    C4d2: Focal C4d staining: 10–50 %
    C4d3: Diffuse C4d staining: >50 %
    Intensity: 1+, 2+, 3+, 4+

Electron Microscopy
The specimen for electron microscopy, studied first by light microscopy with toluidine blue stained one micron thick sections, consists of:

Cores: _____
Composition: cortex, medulla, corticomedullary junction
Number of glomeruli (completely sclerotic): _____
Number of arteries: _____

References

1. Solez K, Colvin RB, Racusen LC, Haas M, Sis B, Mengel M, et al. Banff 07 classification of renal allograft pathology: updates and future directions. Am J Transplant. 2008; 8:753–60.
2. Racusen LC, Solez K, Colvin RB, Bonsib SM, Castro MC, Cavallo T, Racusen, et al. The Banff 97 working classification of renal allograft pathology. 1999;55:713–23.
3. Haas M, Sis B, Racusen LC, Solez K, Glotz D, Colvin RB, et al. Banff 2013 meeting report: inclusion of c4d-negative antibody-mediated rejection and antibody-associated arterial lesions. Am J Transplant. 2014; 14:272–83.

Liver

Liver Transplant Biopsy Evaluation [1]

Acute Cellular Rejection
- **Not present:** Cellular infiltrate within normal limits
- **Indeterminate:** Portal inflammatory infiltrate that fails to meet the criteria for the diagnosis of acute rejection
- **Mild:** Rejection infiltrate in a minority of the triads, that is generally mild and confined within the portal spaces
- **Moderate:** Rejection infiltrate, expanding most or all the triads
- **Severe:** As above for moderate, with spillover into periportal areas and moderate-to-severe perivenular inflammation that extends into the hepatic parenchyma and is associated with perivenular hepatocyte necrosis

Reference

1. Banff schema for grading liver allograft rejection: an international consensus document. Hepatology. 1997;25:658–63.

Small Bowel

Small Bowel Transplant Biopsy Evaluation [1, 2]

- **No ACR:** ≤2 apoptotic bodies per 10 consecutive crypts, no epithelial injury, normal lamina propria
- **Indeterminate for ACR:** 3–5 apoptotic bodies per 10 consecutive crypts, minimal/focal epithelial injury, minimal lamina propria inflammation

- **Mild ACR:** ≥6 apoptotic bodies per 10 consecutive crypts, mild/focal epithelial injury, mild/localized lamina propria inflammation
- **Moderate ACR:** ≥6 or confluent apoptotic bodies per 10 consecutive crypts, focal crypt dropout and focal mucosal erosion, moderate/extensive lamina propria inflammation
- **Severe ACR:** Variable number of apoptotic bodies in residual crypts, extensive crypt dropout with extensive erosion and/or ulceration, moderate to severe and extensive lamina propria inflammation

References

1. Wu T, Abu-Elmagd K, Bond G, Nalesnik MA, Randhawa P, Demetris AJ. A schema for histologic grading of small intestine allograft acute rejection. Transplantation. 2003;75:1241–8.
2. Ruiz P, Bagni A, Brown R, Cortina G, Harpaz N, Magid MS, et al. Histological criteria for the identification of acute cellular rejection in human small bowel allografts: results of the pathology workshop at the VIII International Small Bowel Transplant Symposium. Transplant Proc. 2004;36:335–7.

Limb

Limb Transplant Biopsy Evaluation [1]

Grade 0: No rejection: No or rare inflammatory infiltrates

Grade I: Mild rejection: Mild lymphocytic peri-vascular infiltration. No involvement of the overlying epidermis.

Grade II: Moderate rejection: Moderate to severe peri-vascular inflammation with or without mid epidermal and/or adnexal involvement (limited to spongiosis and exocytosis). No epidermal dyskeratosis or apoptosis.

Grade III: Severe rejection: Dense inflammation and epidermal involvement with epithelial apoptosis, dyskeratosis and/or keratinolysis.

Grade IV: Necrotizing acute rejection: Frank necrosis of the epidermis or other skin structures.

Reference

1. Cendales LC, Kanitakis J, Schneeberger S, Burns C, Ruiz P, Landin L, et al. The Banff 2007 working classification of skin-containing composite tissue allograft pathology. Am J Transplant. 2008;8:1396–400.

Pancreas

Pancreas Transplant Biopsy Evaluation [1, 2]

Acute Cellular Rejection:

Normal	Absent or inactive septal inflammation
Indeterminate for ACR	Active septal inflammation without additional findings, no ductitis or venulitis
Grade I (mild ACR)	Active septal inflammation with ductitis or venulitis and/or 1–2 foci per lobule of acinar inflammation
Grade II (moderate ACR)	Minimal intimal arteritis (<25 % luminal compromise) and/or multiple foci (≥3 foci/lobule) of acinar inflammation with individual cell injury
Grade III (severe ACR)	Diffuse acinar inflammation with focal or diffuse confluent acinar cell necrosis, and/or moderate to severe intimal arteritis; and/or necrotizing arteritis

Acute Antibody-Mediated Rejection:

(Diagnosis requires donor-specific antibodies [DSA], pathologic evidence of tissue injury, and C4d positivity; if only 2 of 3 criteria are present the findings are consistent with AMR; if only 1 criterion is present AMR should be excluded)

Not present

Grade I/mild acute AMR: Well-preserved architecture, mild macrophage or mixed macrophage/neutrophilic infiltrates, rare acinar cell damage

Grade II/moderate acute AMR: Overall preserved architecture, interacinar macrophage or mixed macrophage/neutrophilic infiltrates, capillary dilation, capillaritis, congestion, multicellular acinar dropout, extravasated red blood cells

Grade III/severe acute AMR: Architectural disarray, scattered inflammatory infiltrates with interstitial hemorrhage, multifocal parenchymal necrosis, arterial and venous wall necrosis and thrombosis

Stage of Chronic Rejection:

No significant fibrosis

Stage I (mild graft fibrosis): Fibrosis <30 % of core surface

Stage II (moderate graft fibrosis): Fibrosis occupies 30–60 % of core surface

Stage III (severe graft fibrosis): Fibrotic areas occupy >60 % of the core surface

References

1. Drachenberg CB, Odorico J, Demetris AJ, Arend L, Bajema IM, Bruijn JA, et al. Banff schema for grading pancreas allograft rejection: working proposal by a multi-disciplinary international consensus panel. Am J Transplant. 2008;8:1237–49.
2. Drachenberg CB, Torrealba JR, Nankivell BJ, Rangel EB, Bajema IM, Kim DU, et al. Guidelines for the diagnosis of antibody-mediated rejection in pancreas allografts-updated Banff grading schema. Am J Transplant. 2011;11:1792–802.

UCLA Biopsy Protocols

Heart
- H&E ×3 slides
- Immunostains: CD3, CD20, CD68, C4d and CD68 on first three biopsies and as indicated

Lung
- H&E ×3 slides and trichrome/EVG stain
- GMS and AFB stains if concern for infection

Kidney
- H&E, trichrome, PAS, JMS, H&E, trichrome, PAS, JMS
- IF: C4d and fibrinogen on all biopsies; IgG, IgA, IgM, C1q, C3, albumin, fibrinogen, kappa and lambda if first post-transplant biopsy or concern for glomerular disease or as otherwise indicated
- EM on first post-transplant biopsy or as indicated

Liver
- H&E, trichrome, H&E, PAS, PAS with diastase, H&E, iron
- Additional stains: keratin 7 or 19 to confirm ductopenia, CMV or EBV-EBER, as needed.

Small Bowel
- H&E ×2
- Additional unstained slides for immunohistochemistry or other special stains (adenovirus, CMV, EBV EBER) can be prepared at the time of initial sectioning if clinically indicated

Limb
- H&E ×2 and PAS with diastase and ten unstained slides
- Other stains optional based on H&E findings or for research purposes to include, but not limited to, the following: CD3, CD4, CD8, CD19, CD20, CD68, HLA-DR, CMV, and C4d

Pancreas
- H&E, trichrome, PAS, H&E, trichrome, PAS, H&E
- Additional unstained slides for immunohistochemistry or other special stains (GMS, AFB, C4d, CMV, EBV EBER) can be prepared at the time of initial sectioning if clinically indicated

Index

© Springer International Publishing Switzerland 2016
W.D. Wallace, B.V. Naini (eds.), *Practical Atlas of Transplant Pathology*, DOI 10.1007/978-3-319-23054-2

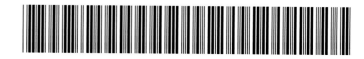